What Every Student Athlete Must Know About Drugs

-The Handbook-

Marvin L. Sims, MSW, CAC

Editor: *Kathleen Gleeson*
Illustrations: *Hans Schmitter*
Cover Design: *Bobbie Russie*
Printed by: *Goodfellow Printing*

ISBN: 0-9634409-1-8

Copyright © 1992 by Marvin L. Sims

Library of Congress Catalog Card Number: 92-96899

All rights reserved. This book is protected by copyright. The reproduction or utilization of this work in any form or by any electronic, mechanical, or other means, including photocopying, recording, and in information retrieval system, is forbidden without written permission from the author.

Printed In The United States of America
10 9 8 7 6 5 4 3 2 1

Additional copies may be ordered from:
   Marvin L. Sims
   1265 Melrose Ave.
   Iowa City, Iowa 52246

For Aaron, LeAnne, Marvin,
Twilla, Forteasha, and Mica,
so that you'll understand the difference.

Contents

Introduction   1
       Drug Facts Test   4

Chapter 1   **Alcohol**   6
       Physical and Mental Effects   6
       Legal Rights/Privileges   9
       Alcohol Use Situations   11
       Sobering Up   12
       Female Athletes and Alcohol   12
       Alcohol Myths   13
       Alcoholism Versus Problem Drinking   14
       Problem Drinking Test   15
       Case Vignette   16

Chapter 2   **Cocaine**   18
       What Is Cocaine   18
       How Cocaine Works   19
       Physical Effects   20
       Case Vignette   20
       Menal Effects   21
       Cocaine and Addiction   22

Chapter 3	**Marijuana**	24
	Case Vignette	24
	What is Marijuana	25
	Hashish	26
	The "Pot" Paradox	26
	Physical and Mental Effects	27
	Medical Uses	28
	Facts and Fictions	29
	Phencyclidine (PCP) and Marijuana	30
	Legal Rights/Privileges	31
Chapter 4	**Anabolic Steroids**	33
	Case Vignette	33
	Why Student Athletes Take Steroids	34
	Steroid Facts	35
	Testosterone	36
	Negative Physical Effects	37
	Females and Steroid Use	38
	Mental Effects	39
	Legal Rights and Privileges	40
Answers To Problem Drinking Test		42
Chapter 5	**Drug Testing**	44
	Intent Of Drug Testing	45
	Body Fluid to be Tested	47
	How Student Athletes Are Tested	47

False Positives and False Negatives	49
Questions Positive Tests Fail to Answer	50
Hair Analysis to Determine Drug Use	50
Diuretics and Drug Testing	50
Sports Organizations That Drug Test	51
NCAA and USOC Testing Policies	51
NCAA and USOC Banned Drugs	52
Who Gets Tested	52
When Test Are Done	52
Penalties For Positive Test	53
NCAA Banned Drug Classes	53
Conclusion	55

Chapter 6 **Human Growth Hormone (hGH)** 58

What is Human Growth Hormone	58
Athletes and hGH	59
How Much Does hGH Cost	59
Negative Health Effects	60
Animal Growth Hormone	61
A Risky Gamble	61

Chapter 7 **Blood Doping and Erythropoietin** 62

Blood Doping	62
What Sports Benefit From Blood Doping	62
How is Blood Doping Performed	62
Adverse Effects	63
Legal Rights and Privileges	64

	Erythropoietin	64
	Medical Uses	64
	Effects on Performance	65
	Adverse Effects	66

Chapter 8 Stimulants — 68
- What are Stimulants — 68
- Why Do Student Athletes Take Stimulants — 68
- **Caffeine** — 69
- **Nicotine** — 70
- Case Vignette — 70
- Smokeless Tobacco — 71
- Physical Effects — 74
- Mental Effects — 75
- School and Team Rules — 76
- **Ephedrine** — 76
- Effects on Performance — 76
- Physical and Mental Effects — 77
- **Amphetamines** — 78
- Medical Uses — 78
- Physical Effects — 78
- Mental Effects — 80
- Effects on Performance — 81
- Legal Right and Privileges — 82

Chapter 9 Depressants — 83
- Clinical Uses — 83

	Effects on Performance	84
	Physical and Mental Effects	85
	Summary	86
Chapter 10	**Reasons, Explanations, Excuses**	87
	Case Vignette	87
	Environment of Exception	89
	Non-Performance Enhancing Drug Use	91
	Stress Producing Factors	91
	Performance Enhancing Drug Use	92
	Factors for Success	93
	Summary	94
Index		96
About the Author		101

List of Tables

1.1	Blood Alcohol Concentrations in Relation to Body Weight	9
2.1	Physical Problems Associated With Cocaine Use	21
2.2	Physical Signs of Cocaine Use	21
2.3	Psychological Problems Associated With Cocaine Use	22
3.1	Behavioral Effects Produced by PCP	31
4.1	Physical Side Effects Experienced by Male Steroid Users	38
4.2	Physical Side Effects Experienced by Female Steroid Users	38
8.1	Banned Over-The-Counter Cold Medicines	77
8.2	Some Physical Complications Associated With Ephedrine Use	77
8.3	Some Mental Complications Associated With Ephedrine Use	77
8.4	Some Negative Side Effects of Amphetamines	79
8.5	Some Ailments Caused by Amphetamine Use	79

Preface

This handbook was written primarily for high school and college students active in sports who want to better understand the complex issues and relationships between drugs and athletics.

It's also necessary reading for parents, administrators, coaches, and sports fans as well.

My concern stems from the misinformation, myths, and falsehoods regarding drugs that student athletes hold to be true. Not understanding the downside and actions of a particular drug (recreational or therapeutic) can lead to unnecessary risk or miscalculation, which in turn can abruptly end an academic and/or athletic career. This handbook is intended to serve as a resource to shed light on many of the performance-enhancing and "street" drug dangers and fallacies.

In our society, drug use and misuse has become an accepted part of everyday life. Drug use and abuse by athletes is a major problem as well. Why do people use drugs? Why would an athlete interested in higher performance voluntarily take something that is known to restrict and even impair physical functioning? These are some of the often asked questions. The objective of this handbook is to provide answers to these questions and give the student athletes facts about drugs to assist them in making informed choices.

Marvin L. Sims

Acknowledgements

I am deeply grateful to Mary Anders who tutored me while I was in graduate school, and who's unremitting assistance during the past few years helped me to attain the skills necessary to undertake and complete this project.

Special thanks go to Tom Davis for the suggestion to develop this book; L. Jay Stein for helping me to understand the laws regarding Driving While Intoxicated (DWI), and Public Intoxication; and to Laura Edgar for the many hours spent in the libraries researching the drug articles and stories of our fallen sports heroes.

Sincere appreciation goes out to Kate Gleeson, editor, for a superb job; and to Hans Schmitter, illustrator, for his cartoons and incredible interpretations of my ideas for drawings.

Introduction

Not many years ago, in 1986, the sports world was shocked and saddened to learn of the sudden death of 22-year-old Len "Frosty" Bias. Len was a consensus All-American for the University of Maryland's basketball team. He was the team's all time leading scorer and the Atlantic Coast Conference Player of the Year both his junior and senior seasons. Bias, a born-again Christian who didn't appear to smoke or drink, averaged 23 points a game his senior year of college, and was the second player selected in the 1986 NBA draft by the Boston Celtics.[1]

Just prior to his NBA rookie season, Len Bias signed a seven-figure shoe endorsement contract with Reebok. While celebrating with friends shortly afterwards, he suffered several of the classic symptoms associated with cocaine overdose: uncontrolled seizures, vomiting, paralysis of breathing muscles, and cardiac arrest. Within a few hours he was dead. Autopsy results showed that Bias's blood cocaine level was 6.5 milligrams per liter, twenty five percent over the lethal concentration level.[2]

Eight days later the tragic scene was performed again when 23-year-old Cleveland Browns safety Don Rogers died from a lethal dose of cocaine on the day before he was to be married. Rogers, an All-American safety at U.C.L.A., averaged over 100 tackles for four seasons, and was the most valuable player in the 1983 Rose Bowl.[3] He was the Brown's first selection in the 1984 National Football

League draft, and he was the American Football Conference defensive rookie of the year.

Rogers had returned to his mother's home after attending a bachelor party given in his honor. The next morning he called out to her, complaining of feeling funny. Rogers had a seizure, collapsed into a coma, and was pronounced dead a few hours later. His heart had stopped. The doctor who performed the autopsy on Rogers found that the lungs and chest cavity of the 6-foot-1-inch, 206-pound star athlete were full of blood: conditions consistent with a drug overdose.[4,5]

You would think that the highly publicized sudden death of Len Bias would have served as a warning to athletes of the world that drugs can kill--even healthy, streetwise, superbly conditioned and trained "super-athletes." Certainly after Don Rogers' death from a lethal dose of cocaine a week later, one would think the message would get around that the risks of drug use are too high. Unfortunately, this is not the case.

Years later not much has changed. Reports of drug use ending the lives and careers of athletes continue to be big news, and the sports world constantly braces itself, fearing a new tragedy at any time. You might think it could never happen to you like that. You figure you'll be smarter, you'll know what to expect, you've got all of the info on drugs. Right? Read on.

Jeff and Mike were returning home from a night of partying downtown following the team's conference championship victory. Jeff dropped Mike off at home and proceeded to his house. Two blocks before he got home, Jeff was stopped by the police. The officer walked over to Jeff's car and asked the young athlete if he knew he had just run a red light. Jeff said he had looked at the light and saw it was green before he went through the intersection. The officer asked Jeff to step outside and take a breathalyzer test which he failed with a .12% blood alcohol level. Jeff was arrested and taken to jail.

Jeff was right in insisting that he thought he saw a green light, and the officer was right in stating that the light was red. How could this be? What Jeff did not know was that alcohol can reduce the sensitivity of the cones in the eyes, making it hard to tell red from green. So the light Jeff saw and thought was green, was actually red.

Did you know alcohol can affect you this way?

In my work, I have often found student athletes to be the most misunderstood individuals on high school or college campuses. As a student athlete you are often in the spotlight, and everyone expects a great deal from you. Your performance and behavior both in and out of your sport produce intense emotional reactions in the general population. You are idolized, resented, revered, and feared. You have your own dreams and fears to contend with, yet far too often you carry the hopes and expectations of your parents, friends, and coaches on your shoulders as well.

You must be prepared to perform and succeed both scholastically and athletically. The time required for each of these undertakings is enormous, and balancing these worlds naturally causes a certain amount of anxiety and tension. In addition, the transitions you undergo from high school to college, from a metropolitan area to a small town, or from a rural to an urban community, can be confusing and difficult. I have observed that this type of adjustment often leads student athletes to experiment with alcohol and other drugs in order to find some relief from uncomfortable situations, thoughts, and pressures. In fact, the major reasons student athletes give me for why they use drugs are to relax, relieve stress, socialize, and belong to the group. They offer other reasons as well: to escape, hide, have a good time, and seek new thrills.

Whatever your motivation, you don't need to become one of the many talented athletes who gets involved in the cycle of drug use and is unable to get out. You don't need to run the risk of ruining your career or your mind because you failed to understand the facts about a particular substance or miscalculated the risk. I am hoping that if you, the student athlete, have more facts about the potential and actual dangers associated with substance use, you will be in a better position to steer clear. Knowing, however, that you still have needs to escape, relax, and belong to the group, I have also included some suggestions to help you meet these needs.

My aim in this handbook is to present the facts: how drugs affect your body, coordination, psyche, rights, and privileges. Let's begin by letting you test your drug intellect so you can get a sense of what you already know and don't know about substance abuse.

Drug Facts Test #1

True or False

1. ____If stopped for suspicion of drinking and driving, you have the legal right to refuse to take a breathalyzer test.
2. ____PCP (Phencyclidine) is a psychedelic powder sprinkled on marijuana to increase its potency.
3. ____One of the most widely prescribed depressant drugs in America today is valium.
4. ____Exercise, drinking black coffee, breathing pure oxygen, or taking a cold shower are good ways to get sober.
5. ____Most drug users make their first contact with illicit drugs through "pushers."
6. ____Human growth hormone (hGH) is the most powerful anabolic steroid known.
7. ____Marijuana is a physically addictive stimulant drug.
8. ____Your driving can be impaired by as little as two drinks of alcohol.
9. ____Addiction to opiates or tranquilizers is a slow process, often taking years to develop.
10. ____Nicotine is a sedative drug present in tobacco.

(Answers on page 42-43)

References

1. Nightingale D: Bias: Shock, Grief, Questions. The Sporting News, June 1986.
2. Dealy Jr. FX: Win at any Cost. The Sell Out of College Athletics. 1990 Birch Lane Press Book, Carol Publishing Group.
3. Browns Safety Dies Of Cardiac Arrest: The New York Times, Saturday, June 28, 1986.

4 Cummings J: Drugs Tied to Rogers Death. The New York Times, Sunday, June 29, 1986.
5 Cummings J: Cocaine Caused Rogers Death. The New York Times, July 1, 1986

Chapter 1

Alcohol

As a student athlete, you undoubtedly know these important facts about alcohol:
1. Alcohol is a drug.
2. Alcohol affects you both physically and mentally.
3. Alcohol is the drug most commonly abused by athletes.
4. Approximately 10%-15% of student athletes who drink "become alcoholics."

You've probably also absorbed some of the myths about alcohol such as "alcohol is a stimulant that makes you high" or "drinking black coffee or taking a cold shower are good ways to get sober."

These facts and myths paint the big picture. Now we're going to zoom in on some of the less familiar, nitty-gritty details that make up that big picture. We'll first look at how alcohol can affect you physically and mentally. Then we'll look at the situations in which student athletes commonly find themselves drinking and consider what other choices or courses of action are available.

PHYSICAL AND MENTAL EFFECTS
Physical Effects

Alcohol acts on your body in two ways: as an irritant and as a sedative.[1] When you drink too much alcohol, it irritates the stomach lining and often produces vomiting. Alcohol can also irritate the pancreas, kidneys, and liver. A healthy liver is critical since it eliminates 90 percent of the alcohol from your bloodstream.

As a sedative, alcohol depresses the central nervous system. The American College of Sports Medicine reports that even a small amount of alcohol--two beers an hour or two prior to competition --can:[2][3]

- slow your reaction time
- impair your hand-eye coordination
- impair muscle reflexes
- disrupt your balance
- diminish your coordination and sense of accuracy

Alcohol also reduces the sensitivity of the cones in your eyes, making it hard for you to tell red from green.

Without mixers, alcohol contains about 200 calories per ounce but has no nutritional value. Since it is nearly empty of essential nutrients such as vitamins and protein, alcohol consumption can result in nutrient imbalance.[4]

One of the long-term effects of alcohol consumption is physical dependence. Dependency steadily deteriorates both training and performance skills. Alcohol is a poison to the human body. Alcohol abuse can lead to organ failure and may cause many life threatening diseases.

The following are long-term health problems caused by alcohol abuse:[5]

- gastrointestinal diseases
- liver damage
- cardiovascular disease
- cancers
- fetal alcohol syndrome
- brain damage

Stay alert and be aware of the dangers of alcohol consumption. Physical dependence on alcohol is a slow process. By the time symptoms develop, serious damage has probably already occurred.

Mental Effects

Alcohol is not a stimulant. It doesn't make you "high" nor does it enhance performance. By depressing your central nervous system, the drug's intoxicating effects often create a false sense of security. As alcohol reaches the brain, it reduces your motivation and diminishes your ability to make proper decisions. Alcohol has consistently been shown to impair information processing. The more rapid reactions your sport requires, the more your performance will suffer.[3]

The age group with the highest percentage of alcohol abuse, 18 to 25, is also the age group of the majority of student athletes. If you drink alcohol, be aware that long-term or chronic use of the drug can lead to psychological dependence. This occurs when alcohol consumption starts to influence or control your daily existence. It is a condition that develops long before symptoms of physical dependence are noticeable. The following are signs of psychological dependence[6]:

1. Self-doubt (doubting your ability to cope without alcohol)
2. Sense of loss (experiencing fear, boredom, and loneliness without alcohol)
3. Inability to abstain from drinking (realizing you can't cope without alcohol)
4. Cravings (relying on alcohol to ease anxiety and tension)
5. Loss of control (caught in a vicious cycle of craving a drink, drinking, and craving more)

The end result of psychological dependence on alcohol is a life-long problem: *alcoholism.*

Legal Rights/Privileges

Blood Alcohol Concentration. If you consume alcohol faster than your body can metabolize it, your Blood Alcohol Concentration (BAC) rises and you become intoxicated. A blood alcohol level of .10 is considered the legal limit for driving a motor vehicle in most states.

Estimated Percentage Of Alcohol In The Blood By Number Of Drinks In Relation To Body Weight

Blood Alcohol Concentrations

Body Wt. Lbs.	1 Drink After Hours 1 / 2 / 3 / 4	2 Drinks After Hours 1 / 2 / 3 / 4	3 Drinks After Hours 1 / 2 / 3 / 4	4 Drinks After Hours 1 / 2 / 3 / 4
100	.043 .028 .013 --	.087 .072 .057 .042	.130 .115 .100 .085	.174 .159 .144 .129
125	.034 .019 .013 --	.069 .054 .093 .024	.103 .088 .073 .058	.139 .124 .109 .094
150	.029 .014 -- --	.058 .043 .028 .013	.087 .072 .057 .042	.116 .101 .086 .071
175	.025 .010 -- --	.050 .035 .020 .005	.075 .060 .045 .030	.100 .085 .070 .055
200	.022 .007 -- --	.043 .028 .013 --	.065 .050 .035 .020	.087 .072 .057 .042
225	.019 .004 -- --	.039 .024 .009 --	.058 .043 .028 .013	.078 .063 .048 .033
250	.017 .002 -- --	.035 .020 .005 --	.052 .037 .022 .007	.070 .056 .040 .025

(-) Means a trace of alcohol

Percent of blood alcohol can be estimated by counting the number of drinks.

1 Drink = 1 ounce whiskey or Vodka, 3 ounces of Wine, or 12 ounces of beer.

Amount of alcohol "burned up" per hour = .015%

Example[7] A 125 lb student who consumes 4 beers in 1 hour has a blood alcohol level of .139%. minus the .015% burned up in the hour = .124%, "legally intoxicated."

(Based on Blood Alcohol Chart, Canada Safety Council)

A breathalyzer test can accurately determine the amount of alcohol in your body. If you are stopped by a law enforcement officer under the suspicion of driving while intoxicated (DWI) but refuse to take a breathalyzer test, you will automatically lose your driver's license for a period of 240 to 540 days. If you not only refuse to take the breathalyzer test but also fail to have a valid driver's license, most states will refuse to issue you a license or permit for the same period a license would be revoked (240-540 days). Driving without a license is punishable by 30 days in jail or a $100.00 fine unless the license has been suspended or revoked, in which case the penalties are more severe.

Public intoxication. Since alcohol is the legal drug that is customarily used in pre-and post-game celebrations, public intoxication is a major cause of concern for many student athletes.

Public intoxication is not a scientifically determined state. The blood alcohol level concentration test used to determine drunken driving or driving while intoxicated is not used in cases of public intoxication. The arresting officer makes a preliminary decision based on subjective observations as to whether or not you were intoxicated, and it's up to the judge and jury to decide whether or not you actually were. The courts look for signs of intoxication such as unusually loud or incoherent speech, an unsteady or staggering gait, and a strong smell of alcohol. In most cases, the arresting officer's testimony is usually enough evidence to convince a judge and jury that you are guilty of the charge.[8] The punishment is usually a fine plus court costs. You and your institution can also receive negative publicity from media accounts of the incident.

Public Drinking. Fewer than half the states have laws against drinking in public. Most states that prohibit public drinking do so in conjunction with a law that bans public intoxication.[7] Before leaving an establishment with alcohol in hand, be sure you know the state laws regulating the public consumption of alcohol.

SITUATIONS

Alcohol before a Contest

As a student athlete you have certainly been warned not to consume alcohol before an athletic contest. However, some misguided athletes drink large amounts of beer prior to a performance in an attempt to load up on carbohydrates (CHO) to fuel their muscles. Alcohol is not a good source of carbohydrates, however. Whereas one 12 ounce glass of juice or an 8 ounce glass of soda contains 40 grams of CHO, one 12 ounce can of regular beer offers only 14 grams of CHO. Light beer has only 5 grams of CHO per 12 ounce serving.[2] You will therefore get much better performance results by drinking fruit juice when trying to increase your carbohydrate levels.

Alcohol after a Contest

I'd be crazy to tell you not to celebrate after a well-deserved victory. But did you know that alcohol is a diuretic, and that diuretics are drugs that increase the rate of urine formation? So instead of satisfying your thirst, alcohol leaves you wanting more to drink. Before rushing off to have a beer after the game, you should first quench your thirst with two or three 12-16 ounce glasses of water to replace sweat loss. Then you should eat some type of carbohydrate (a bagel, muffin, yogurt, or fruit) since carbohydrates delay alcohol absorption better than protein or fat.[2]

Social drinking such as having a beer or two at a "kegger" or post-game party can have negative effects on the well-trained athlete as well.[2] Since alcohol is a sedative, it impairs your judgment, hinders your response time, diminishes your perception and willpower, and slows your mental processing. These detrimental effects can negatively affect your performance for as long as 24 hours.

Many times at post-game parties athletes get involved in "competitive drinking," challenging each other to see who can drink the most. This activity usually results in the consumption of excessive amounts of alcohol and puts the athlete at a very high risk for injury and/or poor decision making such as arguing, fighting, or driving after drinking.

Sobering Up

So okay, against your better judgment you drink too much and need to sober up fast. Unfortunately, contrary to popular belief, you cannot sober up by taking a cold shower, drinking black coffee, or breathing pure oxygen. Exercise does not rid the body of alcohol or help you sober up faster, either.

Alcohol is not stored in the tissues, and less than 10% of the substance is eliminated by sweating. The liver is the chief organ involved in ridding the body of alcohol, and it takes a long time to process the substance. This process is called metabolism. It takes 3 to 5 hours to rid the body of 3 cans of beer, 3 mixed drinks, or 3 glasses of wine.[2] In general, the body eliminates alcohol at a rate of one ounce per hour.

Taking stimulants doesn't make you sober or increase your alertness. It only makes you a drunk who happens to be wide awake.

SOME SPECIAL CASES
Female Athletes and Alcohol

To the female athletes reading this handbook, I should emphasize that alcohol and other drugs pose the same dangers for you as they do for your male counterparts. You, however, have additional issues to be concerned about.

Research has shown that women get drunk slightly faster than men of equal size and weight. This is because women have a significantly smaller amount of an enzyme called *alcohol dehydrogenase* which breaks down alcohol in the stomach.[9] Competitive drinking is therefore particularly unwise if you are a woman since your body may not be able to process alcohol as quickly as you consume it, especially when competing with men.

As females you also need to be aware of the special marketing campaigns designed to get you to increase your alcohol consumption. One of these campaigns involves the marketing of wine coolers. These ads lead you to believe that they are the drink of choice for sophisticated drinkers. By making wine coolers look and taste like soft drinks--some even have straws attached to the boxes--the industry subtly suggests that they are low in alcohol and calories and are non-intoxicating like soft drinks. The fruity, non-alcoholic taste makes it easy for non-drinkers to get started on alcohol, and the shift to drinks with a higher alcohol content becomes less traumatic.

Although effective, this marketing blitz is very deceptive. Brands of wine, beer, and liquor coolers are disguised with juices and syrup to taste like fruit drinks, but most of them have more alcohol than beer or wine; more calories than soda; and, in some cases, "nary a drop of real fruit juice."[10] Wine coolers usually contain 5 to 7 percent alcohol. Most beers average 4 percent.[9]

Wine coolers are shown on television and in other forms of advertising as an alternative to alcohol when having a good time. Don't be fooled. The coolers are not fruit juices or soft drinks; they contain alcohol and can cause the same problems for student athletes as other forms of the drug.

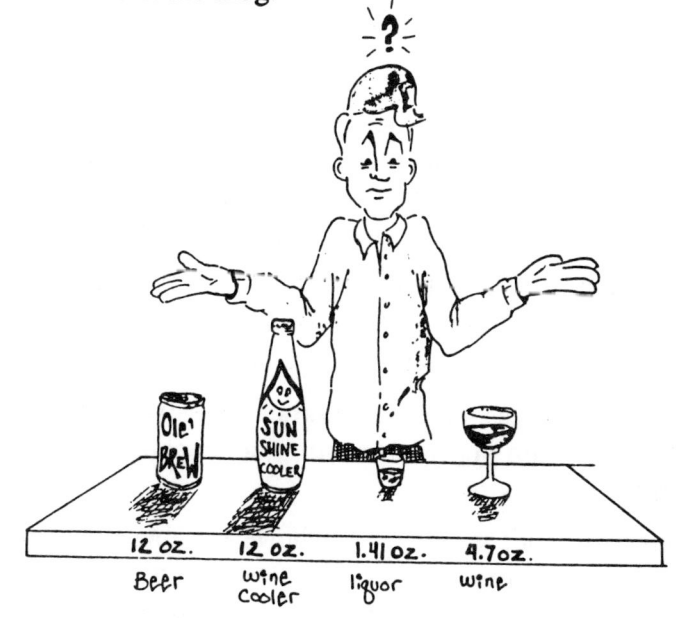

Alcohol Myth

One of the more common myths about alcohol is that beer is less harmful than distilled spirts (whiskey, gin, vodka, rum) and wine.

13

The myth regarding beer's harmlessness is generally due to the misunderstanding of beverage alcohol content. It is true that ounce for once, the alcohol content in distilled spirts is significantly higher than beer or wine. For example, a fifth of 80 proof distilled spirits contains 10.27 ounces of alcohol; a fifth of wine contains 3.08 ounces of alcohol; and a fifth or beer contains 1.21 ounces of alcohol. Looking at it from this perspective it's easy to assume that whiskey is more powerful than beer. [11]

However, "the amount of alcohol contained in each beverage's average [serving] size is precisely the same."[12] 12 ounces of beer contain 0.564 ounces of alcohol, a shot (1.41 ounces) of distilled spirts contain 0.564 ounces of alcohol, and a glass of wine (4.7 ounces) contain 0.564 ounces of alcohol.[11]

The fact is "alcohol is alcohol is alcohol. A can of beer equals a shot of whiskey equals a glass of wine."[13]

Alcoholism Versus Problem Drinking

In my experience, student athletes are rarely alcoholics. Alcoholism is primarily a disease with complex social, genetic, and environmental factors that influence its development. It is usually progressive and often fatal. Typically, alcoholics:

1. Show a preoccupation with alcohol
2. Continue drinking despite obvious adverse consequences
3. Show a pattern of impaired control over drinking
4. Deny their alcohol-related behavior

Fortunately, few student athletes develop an excessive preoccupation with alcohol. Few are <u>unable</u> to control the amount they drink or their frequency of drinking.

A number of student athletes do, however, abuse alcohol and become problem drinkers. In general, student athletes who use alcohol tend to be impulsive drinkers. They tend to be situational drinkers as well, usually choosing not to drink during the playing season. When they do drink they often drink rapidly and excessively, at times with the sole purpose of getting drunk. Even though alcohol use might not immediately affect their ability to perform athletically, it might directly affect their eligibility. Most school policies dictate that an athlete be suspended from team participation for an alcohol-related substance abuse problem.

You can tell that alcohol has become a problem for you when drinking negatively affects your health or upsets your relationships with your family, friends, or teammates, or when it violates the law or school or team rules.

Take a few minutes now to examine your own tendencies and behaviors. If you answer yes to any of the following questions, you could be a problem drinker. If you answer no to all the questions, you're using alcohol responsibly.

Problem Drinking Test #2

1. ____Have you ever awakened in the morning after a night of drinking and found you could not remember part of the evening before?
2. ____Have you ever been arrested or nearly arrested due to alcohol?
3. ____Has anyone close to you (teammate/peer/family) ever been afraid of you or questioned your drinking?
4. ____Do you get drunk more than three times a year?
5. ____Do you use alcohol to help you get through painful situations or feelings?
6. ____Do you drink alone?
7. ____Have you ever felt you ought to cut back on your drinking?
8. ____Have people annoyed you by criticizing your drinking?
9. ____Have you gotten into fights when drinking?
10. ____Have you ever neglected your obligations, family, or class work for two or more days in a row because you were drinking?

(Adapted from the CAGE Questionnaire and The Michigan Alcoholism Screen Test)[14]

Drugs and the Athlete

Bruce Kimball was the 1984 Olympic Silver medalist in platform diving and a six-time national diving champion at the University of Michigan.

16 days prior to the 1988 Olympic trials for which he was favored to qualify, Kimball plowed his car into a group of teenagers on a dark, dead-end street in Brandon, Florida. Two of the youths were killed; another 3 were seriously injured. Kimball admitted he was drunk at the time of the accident. He was arrested and charged with vehicular homicide.[15]

Released on $10,000 bail for the Olympic trials, Bruce tried but failed to make the 1988 Olympic diving team, coming in fourth place. His dives were silently protested by MADD and several friends of the victims.[16] <u>*In February 1989 Bruce was sentenced to 17 years in prison.*</u>

CONCLUSION

Alcohol is the most abused substance on high school and college campuses. Therefore, it is critical that you as a student athlete understand two things: that alcohol is a drug; and that alcohol abuse can cripple or kill you and/or your athletic career.

It's important for you to know that you are responsible for your actions and that there will be consequences for inappropriate behavior displayed while under the influence of alcohol. It is equally important for you to know that there is help available if you need it.

If there is no alcohol information agency available in your area, contact:

> The National Council of Alcoholism
> 12 West 21st Street
> New York, NY 10010
> (212) 206-6770
> (Toll-Free Hotline)1-800-ALCOHOL

Your confidentiality will be protected. Federal law mandates that counselors, psychologists, drug treatment centers, and doctors keep confidential any information received from clients.

References

1. Taylor P: Substance Abuse. Charles C. Thomas, 1988.
2. Clark N: Social Drinking and Athletes, The Physician and Sports Medicine, vol 17 No. 10 Oct. 1989.
3. Position Stand on The Use of Alcohol in Sports. American College Of Sports Medicine 1982.
4. Tabakoff B, Sutker P, Randall C: Medical and Social Aspects of Alcohol Abuse. 1983 Plenum Press, New York.
5. Spence WR: The Medical Consequences Of Alcoholism. 1991 HEALTH EDCO, A Division of WRS Group, Inc., Waco, TX
6. Nace EP: The Treatment of Alcoholism. 1987 Brunner/Mazel, Inc.
7. Wadler GI, Hainline B: Drugs and the Athlete. Philadelphia, F.A. Davis Company 1989.
8. Sloan IJ: Alcohol And Drug Abuse And The Law. 1980 Oceana Publications, Inc.
9. Frezza ET, et al: High Blood Alcohol Levels In Women. The Role of Decreased Gastric Alcohol Dehydrogenase Activity and First-Pass Metabolism. The New England Journal Of Medicine, Vol. 332 No. 2
10. Montgomery A: The Cooler Illusion. Nutrition Action Health Letter, August 1988, p.8.
11. Dealy Jr. FX: Win at any Cost. The Sell Out of College Athletes. Birch Lane Press Book. Carol Published 1990.
12. Dealy, p. 130
13. Alcoholism In The Family: Everybody Trapped by the Bottle? 1990 Krames Communications, San Bruno, CA 94066
14. CAGE Questionaire. The Michigan Alcoholism Screening Test, in Wadler GI, Hainline B: Drugs and the Athlete. Philadelphia, F.A. Davis Company 1989. p. 188-189.
15. Falkner D: Lost Lives, Sheltered Dreams: The Aftermath of a Tragedy. The New York Times, August 22, 1988.
16. Neff C: Diving. Sports Illustrated, August 29, 1988.

Chapter 2

Cocaine

What Is Cocaine?

Few drugs have accumulated so many colorful nicknames: Coke, Girl, Lady, Blow, Toot, and Snow, to list just a few. By any of these names, cocaine is a powerful drug that has a tremendous effect on the central nervous system.

Cocaine is grown on the eastern slopes of the Andes mountains, primarily in Colombia, Bolivia, and Peru. The drug is extracted from the leaves of the coca plant and, when processed, appears as a white powder. On the streets, cocaine is diluted with look-alike substances such as sugar, salt, quinine, strychnine, or other stimulants. Its questionable purity further increases the known dangers associated with cocaine use[1].

Many of you will be told that cocaine is the drug of choice of the elite, rich, powerful, and famous. You'll be told that cocaine will sharpen your instincts, increase your sex drive, and enhance your performance. These stories have been around for years. For a time, cocaine even earned the dubious title "champagne of drugs." People who encourage or dare you to turn onto coke will also tell you it is safe and has no side effects, and that the only people who get hooked are the weak or those who inject it. Don't believe it. This information isn't true. Stories praising the positive effects of cocaine are misperceptions, propaganda, fantasies, and lies.

How Cocaine Works

Cocaine is a local anesthetic that overstimulates the central nervous system. It numbs the mucous membranes and, for a short period of time, tricks the brain into feeling as though it has been supplied with something pleasurable.[1] You experience a feeling of increased energy, alertness, and confidence. This feeling, called a "rush," fades after a very short period of time, approximately 20 to 30 minutes. It is usually followed by feelings of anxiety, irritability, and low mood. Soon thereafter, you experience a strong desire to take more.[1]

Cocaine is highly addictive and has a high potential for abuse. No matter how emotionally well-adjusted you are or how competent, physically fit, and successful in your sport, you are not safe from cocaine's inherent dangers. In fact, most of the known deaths involving athletes and drugs are caused by the use of cocaine.

Cocaine is seductive because it creates a false sense of security or a false sense of enhanced physical skills. Yet no scientific or medical evidence supports the claim that the drug actually enhances athletic performance. On the contrary, cocaine use by athletes has consistently been shown to decrease athletic abilities--and futures.

Baseball players, for example, report having a hard time fielding and hitting the ball while under the effects of cocaine. Pitchers lose something off their fastball and curve, and they report a loss of concentration on the mound. Basketball players lose their shooting touch and become confused during the fast pace of the game. Football players have great difficulty concentrating and following the game plan.[2]

At the college level, sports recruiters listen for reports of drug use by prospective high school recruits. Because of its high addiction potential, the first drug they worry about is cocaine. In professional sports, an athlete's drug history has become one of the major variables when college draft or trade talks get started. As much time is now spent learning an athlete's drug history as is spent studying his or her ability to perform. The first question club owners now ask about a prospect is "Is this athlete healthy and clean?"[3]

PHYSICAL AND MENTAL EFFECTS

Physical Effects

Cocaine increases blood pressure, body temperature, and heart-rate. All of these symptoms can overstimulate and stress the heart.

The major health risk associated with cocaine use is sudden death. Sudden death usually results from "uncontrolled seizures, paralysis of breathing muscles, irregularities of heartbeat, or cardiac arrest."[4] Death can result from ingesting as little as 1 to 2 lines of the drug and can occur so quickly that there is no time to get medical help.[5]

Cocaine use can also cause nutrient imbalance since the drug suppresses the appetite, often to the point of vitamin deficiency and anorexia.

Drugs and the Athlete

On October 11, 1988 David Croudip, a 29-year-old defensive back with the Atlanta Falcons, was rushed to Joan Glancy Hospital in Duluth, Georgia after suffering a seizure at home.

Croudip, a defensive back and captain of special teams, had started his professional football career in the United States Football League (USFL) in 1983 with the Los Angeles Express and moved to the National Football League in 1984 when he signed on with the Los Angeles Rams. In 1985 Croudip had a short stint with the San Diego Chargers before signing on with the Falcons.

On this fated day, Croudip returned home shortly after losing a football game to the Los Angeles Rams. He fixed himself a drink of juice or water laced with cocaine to pick himself up for the evening. Rather than feel more alert and energized, David Croudip had a seizure and was pronounced dead at 3:30 am.

<u>The death was caused by an overdose of cocaine ingested in one dose.</u> Croudip had always tested negative for the presence of drugs in the National Football League (N.F.L) drug screening program.[6,7]

Table 2.1

Physical Problems Associated with Cocaine Use

1. Chronic Insomnia
2. Nasal & Sinus Infections
3. Severe Headaches
4. Convulsions
5. Heart Attacks
6. Chronic Fatigue
7. Disrupted Sexual functioning
8. Increased blood pressure
9. Tremors

Table 2.2

Physical Signs of Cocaine Use [8]

1. Extreme loss of body weight
2. Nasal septum irritation
3. Convulsions
4. Intense itching in the limbs
5. Tired or blurry eyes
6. Persistent hacking cough with dark sputum

Mental Effects

Cocaine is a mood-altering drug that has a profound effect on the psyche. It produces a distorted sense of time, slows reaction and timing, and severely affects judgment.

Initial use of cocaine causes feelings of euphoria and self-confidence. It produces a distorted sense of self and reality. Your fears and stresses seem to lessen. You think you can run faster, jump higher, react quicker, and see better. You feel you can do anything and everything.

Consistent use of cocaine causes athletes to undergo personality changes. Continued use over time, either sporadically or frequently, causes behavior to become erratic. Loyalty and team responsibility lose their importance. Your work and study habits, ethics and attitudes, change as the drug becomes more and more important, and your athletic skills steadily deteriorate.

Table 2.3
Psychological Problems Associated with Cocaine Use

1. Depression	6. Decreased concentration
2. Paranoia	7. Loss of non-drug using friends
3. Anxiety	8. Loss of interest in non-drug
4. Irritability	related activities

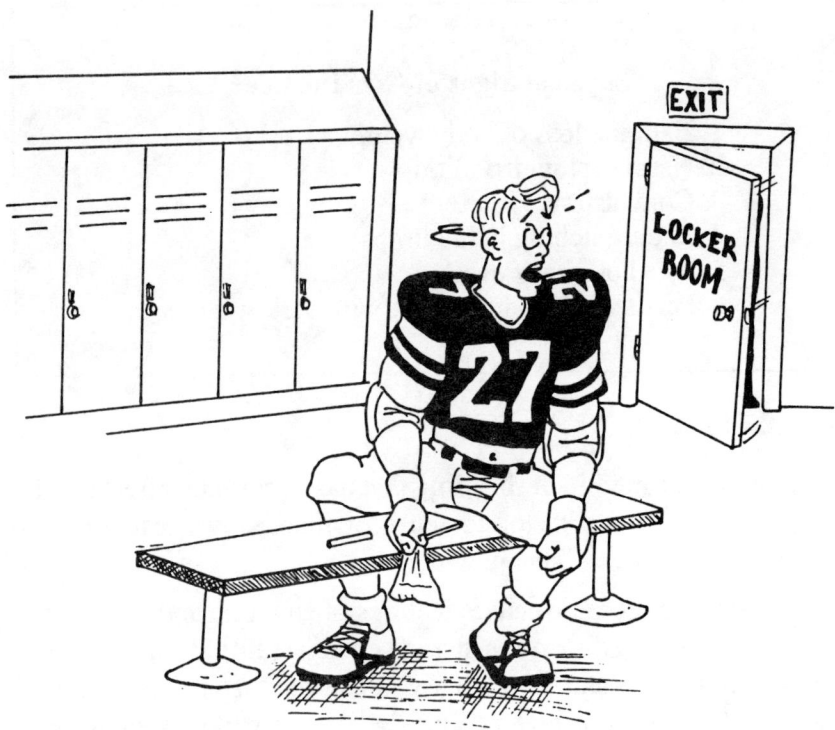

Cocaine Is Addictive

Make no mistake, regardless of how much hype you hear or how glamorized the drug seems, cocaine is highly addictive. Some people become addicted the first time they try it while others take from weeks to months to become dependent.

Cocaine is powerfully addicting because its intensely pleasurable effects are immediate. However, due to the liver's metabolism, the high only lasts for a brief period of time. To recreate the euphoric feelings, the user is driven to take more of the drug. Repeated use establishes a tolerance level so that it takes more cocaine to get the desired results.

When the effects begin to wear off, negative feelings such as low mood, fear, and irritability replace the good, pleasant feelings. These negative feelings are just as strong as the positive feelings. To get rid of them, the user experiences a strong urge to take more of the drug. Giving in to this drive puts you firmly on the path to addiction.

References

1. Spence WR: Cocaine, The Unseen Dangers. HEALTH EDCO, WRS Group Inc. Waco TX.
2. Kirkman D: Experts: Coke even hurts best athletes. Newsday, April 24, 1986.
3. Murray C, Goodwin M: Cocaine Disrupts Baseball From Field to Front Office. The New York Times, August 20, 1985.
4. Washton A, Gold M, et al: Cocaine: A Clinicians Handbook. 1987 The Guilford Press, New York.
5. Washton, p. 24.
6. Schwartz J: Falcon Player Dies at Age 29. The New York Times, October 11, 1988.
7. Sports People: Clearly, an overdose. The New York Times, October 13, 1988.
8. Allen D, et al: The Cocaine Crisis, 1987 Plenum Press, New York.

Chapter 3

Marijuana

Jason, a 21-year-old student athlete, had just completed his senior football season and went out to celebrate with friends. Some people were smoking marijuana at a party, and they asked Jason to join in. He had always been curious about pot but had resisted the temptation to try it because it was against the athletic department and team rules.

However, since a very successful season and college football career were over, Jason was in a good mood and felt this was the time to satisfy his curiosity about marijuana. He smoked some weed from a bong with a few friends and sat back to enjoy the evening.

Approximately 30 minutes later, Jason realized he was getting too deeply into his thoughts. He couldn't say exactly how, but he realized he was having trouble changing his focus or topic of conversation. He felt as though he knew all of the people around him, but he didn't know who he was. Jason panicked and left the party. He headed back to the dorm, afraid of the people he saw on the street.

Jason went to bed when he got to his room but couldn't fall asleep. He tried desperately to vomit, but nothing came up. Jason then experienced a falling sensation, as though he were falling into a large bottomless pit. He was sure he was going to die but still didn't know who he was.

More afraid than he had ever been in his life, Jason gathered himself together, walked to the hospital emergency room, and admitted himself. The nurses and doctors helped him to relax and ran several tests. One test came back positive for THC (marijuana).

Did you know that marijuana can impair short-term memory or affect your body and senses in this way?

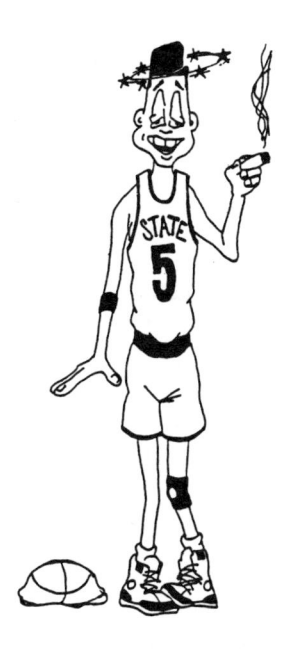

What is Marijuana?

Marijuana is a mood-altering drug commonly referred to as pot, reefer, grass, or weed. It grows wild in many parts of the United States and around the world. The greenish brown mixture is made from the dried leaves, seeds, stems, and flowers of the hemp plant. The hemp plant, *cannabis sativa*, is known to have been used by the Chinese thousands of years ago for weaving. However, by 100 B.C. the Chinese had discovered the plant's mind-altering qualities and began using the juice to provide psychic pleasures.[1]

With over 400 chemical entities in the plant (approximately 60 are biologically active), marijuana is a very complicated drug.[1] Its main psychoactive component is THC (tetrahydrocannabinol). Due to its sedative properties, THC is commonly known as a central nervous system depressant. However, this is only half the truth because THC can stimulate the central nervous system as well.

The smoke contained in one marijuana cigarette contains approximately 6 mg of THC.[2] The effects of THC vary from individual to individual. The reactions can be different for each person and can be different each time it's used. Many internal and external factors over which you have little or no control determine your response to smoking pot.

What is Hashish?

Hashish, also known as hash, is a concentrated form of marijuana made from the dark brown resin collected from the tops of the cannabis plant. The plants are harvested and dried, then compressed into many forms such as cakes, balls, or loaves.

The percentage of THC in hashish is approximately five times greater than that in regular marijuana. Therefore, the effects of the drug are more intense and unpleasant side effects are more likely.[3]

The Pot Paradox

Marijuana has no performance-enhancing qualities, yet it is the most widely used illicit drug by student athletes. Following alcohol and tobacco, marijuana is America's third drug of choice.

Although not physically addicting, marijuana has been shown to be highly psychologically addicting. Psychological addiction is a slow process that usually starts with experimentation or casual use. The frequency of use increases gradually until the drug becomes a regular part of life.

When you're high on pot your problems don't seem as bad as when you're "straight." You deal with stress better. You have more fun. You realize that you're able to do and say things when high that you normally wouldn't do or say. Smoking pot, then, becomes your crutch or way to deal with disappointment and unpleasant situations. You begin to believe you can't cope with the activities of daily life without it. You are now psychologically addicted.

PHYSICAL AND MENTAL EFFECTS

Physical Effects

Although marijuana is usually known as a psychologically addicting drug, it may also cause physical health problems and complications. Smoking pot can speed up your heart rate and raise your blood pressure as much as 50 percent, depending on the amount and potency of THC you consume. Marijuana contains up to 50 percent more tar than cigarettes as well as many other cancer-causing chemicals.[4]

Marijuana interferes with the lung's pumping and filtering action which in turn decreases the oxygen flow. It impairs hand-eye coordination, slows reaction time, and impairs visual tracking abilities. Like alcohol, marijuana can produce a next day hangover.[4]

Other physical side effects of marijuana include: [4]

> a decrease in hormones that control sexual growth and development
>
> decreased sperm production in males
>
> disruption of the female menstrual cycle
>
> depression of the immune system

Recent reports reveal that prolonged marijuana use can lower the testosterone levels in men and increase the levels in women. Sufficient testosterone levels are critical for the development and maintenance of male sexual characteristics. Overproduction of testosterone in women can decrease female sexual characteristics and lead to the development of male sexual characteristics. [3]

Mental Effects

Marijuana has various psychological effects on its users. It can distort your perception of time and space as well as your hearing and vision. Initially, you feel as though your ability to think and reason have been enhanced. However, eventually you find that you can grossly misinterpret sensations and events and experience non-existent sensations.[5]

The drug produces a lapse in judgment, causes difficulty in concentration, and decreases memory, reasoning, coordination, and intellectual functioning. Marijuana can cause the brain to perceive time to move slower than it actually is (altered perception of time). This perception can adversely affect athletic performance or cause injury.[1]

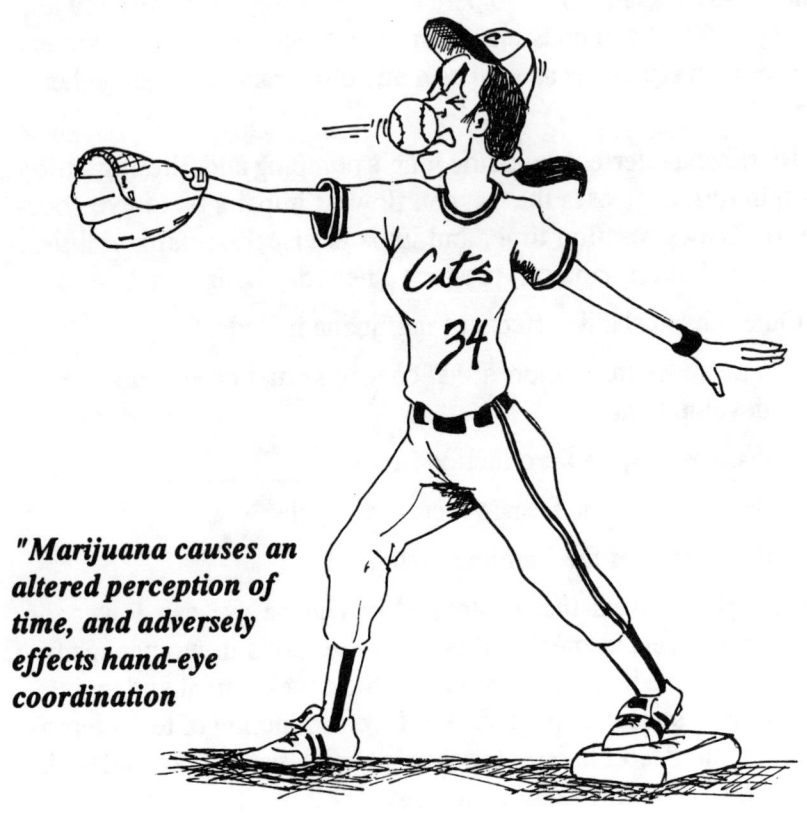

"Marijuana causes an altered perception of time, and adversely effects hand-eye coordination

Medical Uses

Marijuana has been researched for many years. Several medical applications have been found for the drug:[2]

1. Prevention of nausea and vomiting in patients receiving chemotherapy
2. Use as a bronchodilator in patients with asthma
3. Treatment of some convulsive disorders
4. Reduction of fluid pressure in the eyes

MARIJUANA FACTS AND FICTIONS

FICTION: Marijuana is a harmless recreational drug.

FACT: *Marijuana is generally known as a depressant and mood-altering drug with many health risks. Marijuana can cause psychological addiction.*

FICTION: The effects of pot last only an hour or so.

FACT: *The high from pot is felt in minutes, reaches its peak in 20-30 minutes, and fades in an hour or two. After this period of time you may feel normal or in control, but the drug can continue to impair judgment, concentration, and coordination for 24 hours or more.*

FICTION: Smoking marijuana leads to a higher awareness of self and others.

FACT: *Marijuana smokers are more likely to isolate themselves from teammates, friends, and family members. When you're high on pot you let the world pass by and withdraw into yourself. You escape from everyday life, seeing neither yourself nor those around you realistically.*

FICTION: The coach or teachers will know if a student athlete is having problems due to marijuana use.

FACT: *Signs of trouble or dependence are hard to spot in the early stages. Marijuana produces different reactions in different people. The response you get depends on the drug's potency, your personality, your frame of mind prior to use, and many other factors.*

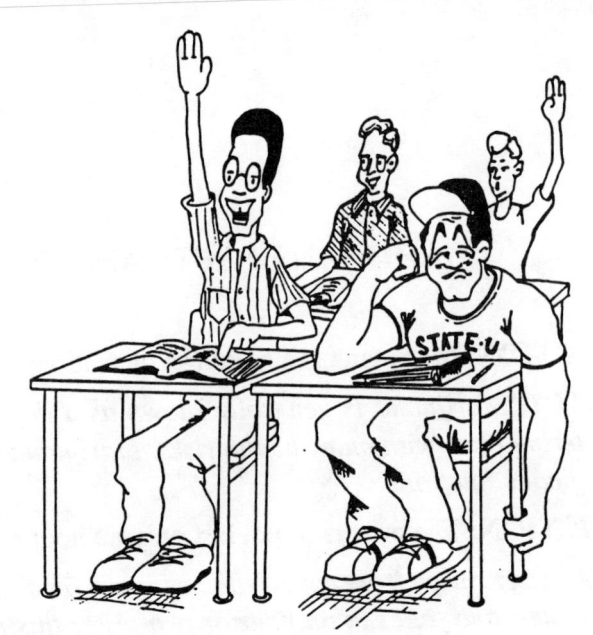

Marijuana continues to impair judgment, concentration and coordination long after the effects of the high have faded.

PCP (Phencyclidine) and Marijuana [26]

PCP is a synthetic hallucinogenic drug that, in its pure form, appears as a white crystalline powder. However, most PCP is made in secret laboratories and contains contaminants, so the color usually ranges from tan to brown.

PCP can be taken orally, intravenously, or "snorted " (inhaled through the nasal passages). However, generally the drug is sprinkled on parsley leaves, mint, or marijuana and smoked. *A common practrice among drug dealers is to lace weak batches of pot with PCP.*

For a brief period in the 1960s, doctors used PCP as a surgical analgesic and anesthetic. In 1965 the drug was banned from use in humans due to its side effects such as agitation, confusion, and delirium.

From 1967 to 1978 PCP was marketed for use in veterinary medicine. During this same time period, the drug began appearing on the black market under names such as Angel Dust, Crystal, WAC, Embalming Fluid, Super Weed, Rocket Fuel, and THC. These oddball names are said to accurately reflect the drug's bizarre and unpredictable effects.

Table 3.1
Behavioral Effects Produced by PCP[2,6]

a sense of detachment	loss of coordination
floating sensations	severe mood swings
auditory hallucinations	intense blank stares
involuntary eye movements	slurred or blocked speech

sense of strength and invulnerability
feelings of sensory or emotional isolation
distorted body images as in a fun-house mirror

PCP is a powerful psychedelic that poses a greater risk to the user than other drugs.[2] Aggressive and violent behavior while on PCP is common. So is arrest by the police, accidents, and death. PCP is the ultimate Bad Trip.

Legal Rights/Privileges

Marijuana is on the banned substances list of the National Collegiate Athletic Association (NCAA) and is listed as a street drug along with heroin and THC. However, marijuana is not banned by the International Olympic Committee (IOC) or the United States Olympic Committee (USOC).[1] Despite the conflict in policies, you should keep in mind that marijuana is an illegal drug in the United States (except Alaska) and possession of the substance is punishable by a fine, jail term, or both.

References

1. Wadler GI, Hainline B: Drugs and the Athlete. Philadelphia, F.A. Davis Company 1989.
2. Taylor P: Substance Abuse. Charles C. Thomas, 1988.
3. Spence WR: Marijuana: How Much Of A Gamble? 1991 HEALTH EDCO, A Division of WRS Group, Inc., Waco TX.
4. Dye C: Marijuana-Health Effects. February 1988 D.I.N Publication, Phoenix, AZ.

5. Sloan IJ: Alcohol And Drug Abuse And The Law. 1980 Oceana Publications, Inc.
6. Drugs Of Abuse: 1988 United States Department Of Justice Publication. Drug Enforcement Administration, Washington, D.C.

Chapter 4
Anabolic Steroids

Drugs and the Athlete

Angel Myers was projected to be one of the United States top medal winners in the 1988 Olympics. As a freshman at Furman University, she set NCAA Division II swimming records in the 100-yard freestyle, 200-yard individual medley, and the 100-yard butterfly. She also won the 50-yard freestyle event at the national championship.[1]

On the opening day of the 1988 United States Olympic swimming trials in Austin, Texas, Myers, a 21-year old college junior, set two American swim records. She set the women's 100-meter freestyle event twice. In the morning prelims she beat the old record of 55.30 when she was clocked at 55.15. In the finals she smashed the record again with a time of 54.95. She then broke Dara Torre's American record (25.59) in the 50-meter freestyle finals with a time of 25.40.[2] *In all, Myers qualified for five events at the 1988 Olympic trials and was talented enough to win medals in all five.*[3]

Following the Olympic trials the "powerfully built," 5' 5", 145-pound Myers tested positive for anabolic steroids and was removed from the United States Olympic swim team. Angel denied taking any banned substances and appealed the suspension, claiming the test had mistakenly identified birth-control pills as evidence of steroid use.[4]

A three member United States Olympic Committee (USOC) arbitration panel met to address the appeal, and Angel testified before the panel. On September 2, 1988, the deadline date for United States Olympic team certification, the panel upheld Myers removal from the team. [4]

WHY DO STUDENT ATHLETES TAKE STEROIDS?

to get stronger	to impress peers
to build muscle	to earn college scholarships
to be competitive	to look "macho"

professional contracts

Anabolic steroids were once seen as a drug that only competitive male weightlifters and professional body builders used. The drugs were primarily used in sports requiring strength, massive muscles, explosiveness, and stamina. Today, male and female athletes alike take the drugs. Steroid use is seen in track and field events, hurdling, swimming, cycling, distance and sprint running, boxing, softball, tennis, and football. It is estimated that as many as 400,000 teenagers now use steroids. This compares to an estimate of 260,000 teen users four years ago.[5] The escalated use of steroids by student athletes on high school and college campuses has created serious health and ethical concerns for athletes, coaches, and competitive sports in general.

Suspicion and competitive paranoia surrounding steroids has escalated through the years. Athletes participating in elite athletic competitions at the international level and increasingly more in college and high school sports ask, "Is the drug-free athlete a losing athlete?" Many competitors think so.

Paranoia about steroid use perpetuates a feverous competitive state. Many student athletes begin to use them for fear of not being able to perform at the same level as their teammates or competitors. However, the impression that all student athletes are using steroids is false, for the great majority of you are not.

In an attempt to address this problem, the National Collegiate Athletic Association (NCAA) started post-season drug testing in 1986. Following the first testing period, more than 20 collegiate athletes from at least seven universities, including former Oklahoma University and Seattle Seahawks linebacker Brian Bosworth, were barred from post-season bowl games due to positive tests for steroid use.[6] Canadian sprinter Ben Johnson was forced to return his gold medal after testing positive for the anabolic steroid stanozolol following his record breaking 100-meter dash (9.79 seconds) at the 1988 Olympic Summer Games. Two Bulgarian weight lifters were also stripped of their medals. A total of ten positive drug tests were reported at the 1988 Olympic Games in Seoul, South Korea.[7] A New York Times report estimated that of the 9,000 athletes who competed, 50 percent of them were on drugs.[8]

Since the highly publicized account of Ben Johnson's rise and tragic fall from glory, reports of steroid use and abuse among high school, college, and elite athletes have become commonplace. Teenage boys and girls are now using steroids not only to enhance their athletic performances but to gain peer approval, bolster self-esteem, and improve appearance.

DID YOU KNOW?

A report in the Journal of the American Medical Association revealed that 6.6% of male high-school seniors and perhaps as many as 500,000 adolescents nationwide have used steroids.[9]

A Northeastern University study by the Center for Study of Sport in Society found 36% of high-school athletes knew someone who had used steroids.[10]

The Inspector General's Office conducted a study which showed that more than a quarter-million of all adolescents in grades 7-12 use or have used steroids.[10]

How much do you really know about these mysterious hormones? Do you know that not all steroids are anabolic or tissue building? A group of steroids known as *corticosteroids* are anti-inflammatory and anti-asthmatic hormones prescribed by doctors to treat conditions such as bursitis, phlebitis, asthma, and emphysema.

Anabolic steroids are hormones that naturally occur in the human body, specifically as testosterone and its derivatives. The term anabolic means tissue building. Since these hormones are also masculinizing or androgenic they are called anabolic-androgenic steroid hormones.[11] Testosterone can also be artificially created in labs. These manufactured anabolic steroids are referred to on the streets as Juice or Roids.

Testosterone, a hormone necessary for muscle development, occurs naturally in large quantities in men but only in small amounts in women (approximately 100 times less).[12] In men, testosterone is primarily produced in the testicles. A much smaller amount of the hormone is produced by the adrenal glands. In women, the primary source of testosterone is the adrenal glands.[13]

Testosterone triggers the following masculine changes that occur in males during puberty: [11]

- lowering of voice
- growth of body hair
- maturation of the penis and testicles
- production of sperm
- broadening of the shoulders
- development of sex drive
- development of aggressiveness

The controversy surrounding anabolic steroid use has been complicated by the fact that for many years athletic trainers, coaches, physicians, and sports medicine officials told athletes that the drugs did not enhance muscle size and strength and that they had many potentially harmful effects. The positive effects of steroids was denied to try and maintain sports purity and equality. Officials thought that if they said the drugs didn't work, then athletes wouldn't try them. Athletes using the drugs could see, however, that the drugs significantly enhanced muscle size, power, and athletic performance. Consequently, they disregarded the entire message, refusing to listen to or believe the doctors and educators when told about the drugs potentially dangerous side effects. This mixed message has cost the medical profession credibility with athletes.[7]

In order to combat this menacing problem, the deception must end. **STEROIDS DO WORK**. Anabolic steroids can enhance athletic ability if the athlete is "concurrently ingesting adequate dietary protein and calories and undergoing intensive weight training." [14]

Negative Physical Effects

Steroids work, but they have many real and potentially negative health consequences. The following physical side effects occur in males:

Stunting of growth. Steroid use by teenagers can be especially dangerous. A student athlete trying to make the squad or earn a starting position on the team might be tempted to use the drugs to build muscles and get stronger. If the youngster hasn't reached full height, the use of steroids can close the growth plates at the ends of bones sooner than normal. In addition, leg and arm cartilage may prematurely turn into bone and stunt bone growth.[10]

Increase in ligament and tendon injuries. Anabolic steroids have been known to increase muscle size and strength before the tendons, joints, and connective tissue have had a chance to develop. This increases the susceptibility of injuring connective and supportive tissue."[15]

Gynecomastia (breast-growth). Gynecomastia, the swelling of the nipple area and development of breast tissue in men,[14] is one of the verified effects of male steroid usage. It appears as a tender mass of tissue under one or both breasts.[10] Plastic surgery is often needed to correct this condition.

Testicular Atrophy (shrinking of the testicles). Synthetic testosterone introduced into the body can confuse your system and cause the testicles to produce and circulate less of the natural hormone. This can lead to many side effects such as testicle shrinkage and decreased sperm production. It can also lead to impotence and sterility.

For all student athletes there is an *increased cancer risk* associated with the use of anabolic steroids. The body's natural defense system is tied to hormonal balance. When steroids are introduced into this delicate balance, many hormone changes occur. When that balance is altered or weakened, cancer cells can more easily develop and reproduce.

Table 4.1

Other Physical Side Effects Experienced by Male Steroid Users :

Premature hair loss
Severe acne
Increased risk of liver and kidney abnormalities
Increased risk of cardiovascular problems
Elevated cholesterol levels
Increase in blood pressure
Increased irritability and aggressiveness
Increased sex drive
Urinary hesitancy

Female student athletes who take anabolic steroids will experience a *masculinizing effect.* This is because the differences in secondary sexual characteristics between males and females are determined by testosterone.[10] Steroid use by females is more hazardous than it is for males because females normally have significantly less testosterone in their systems. Therefore, taking steroids adversely effects the system of glands that regulate female body functions. This system is called the "endocrine gland loop" and includes the pituitary, thyroid, adrenal glands, and ovaries.[11]

Table 4.2

Physical Side Effects Experienced by Female Steroid Users:

Permanent deepening of the voice	Decreased breast size
Cessation of menstrual periods	Premature hair loss
Increased sex drive	Increased body and facial hair
Increased risk of kidney damage	Urinary hesitancy
Severe acne	Enlarged clitoris
Increased aggressiveness	Elevated blood pressure
Elevated cholesterol level	Liver and breast abnormalities

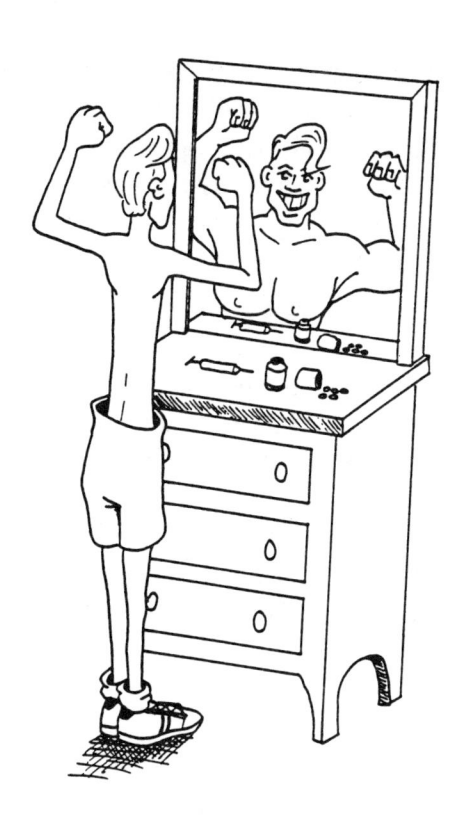

Mental Effects

Undoubtedly, the use of anabolic steroids can affect the mind dramatically. Your body image and self-concept may become severely distorted (the reverse of anorexia nervosa) as you become obsessed with building muscle.

Many steroid users report experiencing a "rush" or "natural high" when on a "roid" cycle. They become more assertive and have an inflated sense of self-worth. Many athletes' self-image is based on how they look and how much weight they can lift. A powerful self-image that has been shaped through the use of steroids is very difficult to change. Once on the drugs it's extremely hard to get off.

When you stop taking steroids, your body's normal level of testosterone cannot sustain the huge muscles and increased strength. Size disappears fast. The gained strength and increased lifts on the weights go down as your body adjusts. You lose approximately 25% of whatever muscle mass you gained very quickly. Shortly thereafter, your body returns to normal. As your size shrinks, so do your feelings of power, machoism, and invincibility. You may then begin to feel insecure and experience mood swings and listlessness. You can often become depressed. To counter the symptoms of depression and the negative self-image brought on by the loss of strength and body size, many steroid users return to the cycle. They are then on the troubled road of *psychological addiction.*

Another classic side effect associated with steroid use is *increased aggressiveness.* Heightened assertiveness, hostility, and irritability are commonly reported symptoms. Although this upsurge in aggression may be beneficial in training and in some sporting events, the aggressive tendencies are difficult to control and are usually undesirable during everyday life. Since steroid users are likely to become combative, impatient, and moody, interpersonal problems often occur such as "fights with other athletes, girlfriends, strangers, or walls."[16]

Legal Rights/Privileges

In November 1990, a new federal law was passed prohibiting the possession, prescription, and distribution of anabolic steroids for use in humans other than for the treatment of diseases or other medical conditions. This law is called the Anabolic Steroids Control Act (ASCA). Its primary objective is to eliminate the sale of anabolic steroids through the black market since this is where approximately 75 percent of all steroid sales occur.

The law categorizes anabolic steroids as Schedule III drugs. This category includes drugs or other substances that are currently accepted for use in medical treatment in the United States, yet have a potential for abuse. Use of Schedule III drugs may lead to moderate physical dependence or high psychological dependence.

Penalties. First offense can carry a prison sentence of up to 5 years and fines of up to $250,000. A second offense can bring 10 years in prison and fines of up to $500,000.[17]

Student athletes who take anabolic steroids want larger muscles and a quick route to recognition. However, the physical and mental problems associated with steroid abuse far outweigh the increases in peer status, strength, and muscle mass.

In the athletic arena, there are no quick fixes or magic potents. If you are thinking about shortcuts, think again about the high price your body and mind will pay. Is it really worth it?

References

1. Faces In The Crowd: Angel Myers. Sports Illustrated, April 21, 1986.
2. Neff C: Back To The Future. Sports Illustrated August 22, 1988.
3. Notebook: U.S. Committee Closes Book on Myers. The New York Times. Sunday September 18, 1988.
4. Sports People: Myers Appeal Fails. The New York Times. Saturday, September 18, 1988.
5. Kuznik F: The Steroid Epidemic. USA Weekend, May 15-17, 1992.
6. Medical News and Perspectives: Steroids in Sports: After Four Decades, Time to Return These Genies to Bottle? JAMA, January 23/30, 1987-Vol 257, No. 4.
7. Cowart VS: Medical News and Perspectives: Accord on Drug Testing, Sanctions Sought Before 1992 Olympics in Europe, JAMA, December 16, 1988-Vol 260, No. 23.
8. Dealy Jr. FX: Win at any Cost. The Sell Out of College Athletics. 1990 Birch Lane Press Book, Carol Publishing Group
9. Toufexis A: Shortcut to the Rambo Look. Time Magazine, January 30, 1989.
10. Jackson LM: Schools fight steroids' grip on students. USA Today, November 19, 1990.
11. Strauss RH: Anabolic Steroids: Drugs and Performance In Sports. W.B. Saunders Company 1987.
12. Groves D: The Rambo Drug. American Health. September 1987.
13. Taylor WN: Anabolic Steroids and the Athlete. McFarland and Company, Inc., 1982.
14. Taylor, p. 3.
15. Almond E, Cart J, Harvey R: Choosing Sides on Steroids. LosAngeles Times, Tuesday, January 31, 1984.
16. Strauss, p. 63.
17. Ramotar JE: Geting tougher on steroid abuse. The Physician and SportsMedicine, vol 19 No. 2, February 1991.

Drug Smart Test #1--(Answers)

1. If stopped for suspicion of drinking and driving, you have the legal right to refuse to take a breathalyzer test.

    (True) You have a legal right to refuse to take a breathalyzer test, but if you do, you will automatically lose your driver's license.

2. PCP (Phencyclidine) is a psychedelic powder sprinkled on marijuana to increase its potency.

    (True) One of the all too common practices of "pushers" and drug dealers is to lace their weak batches of pot with PCP. This illicit drug can produce unpredictable, erratic, and violent behavior in users. These actions can be directed at themselves or at others.

3. One of the most widely prescribed depressant drugs in America today is valium.

    (True) Valium is one of the top five most prescribed drugs in America and has been for many years.

4. Exercise, drinking black coffee, or taking a cold shower are good ways to get sober.

    (False) There are no shortcuts to sober a drunk person. Once alcohol is in the bloodstream it takes time for the body to rid itself of the substance. This process, called metabolism, takes about one hour for each drink taken.

5. Most drug users make their first contact with illicit drugs through "pushers."

    (False) The first contact is usually through their friends. The pressure from friends to experiment with drugs can influence many people to start using drugs.

6. Human growth hormone (hGH) is the most powerful anabolic steroid known.

    (False) Human growth hormone is not a steroid. hGH is a hormone produced by the pituitary glands.

7. Marijuana is a psychologically addictive stimulant drug.

> *(False)* *Although marijuana is psychologically addicting, it is a depressant, not a stimulant.*

8. Your driving can be impaired by as little as two drinks of alcohol.

> *(True)* *Driving is impaired at blood alcohol levels as low as .05%. Depending on your body weight and metabolism, you can reach that level with as little as two drinks.*

9. Addiction to opiates or tranquilizers is a slow process and often takes years to develop.

> *(False)* *Unlike addiction to alcohol, which can take years to develop, you can become addicted to opiates or tranquilizers in a matter of weeks.*

10. Nicotine is a sedative drug present in tobacco.

> *(False)* *Nicotine, a potent drug found in smoking and smokeless tobacco, is a central nervous system stimulant.*

Chapter 5

Drug Testing

Among student athletes, the hottest and most controversial topic is drug testing. Many student athletes believe drug testing is an infringement on their human and civil rights, and many civil libertarians agree with this position. Test validity and fairness are hotly debated when the subject is raised.

It's important for you to know that unless it is an emergency situation, informed voluntary consent must be obtained when performing urine tests on any person 18 years of age or older.[1] If you are a high school athlete, you should be aware of the ethical and legal implications involved in performing urine tests on minors. Drug testing on minors is an issue that must be resolved by either a physician or the courts. Due to the potential for costly legal problems, drug education is the approach normally used by most community and high school sports organizations.

One exception to the rule is the policy set forth by the East Chambers Independent School District in Winnie, Texas. In 1988 this district of 500 students began random drug testing and drug education programs for all students in the sixth grade and above who participated in extracurricular activities. The program tests for drugs of abuse including cocaine, marijuana, amphetamines, and anabolic steroids. Urinalyses are performed during school hours and the results are confidential. Students who test positive are suspended from all extracurricular activities for a specified period of time,[2] although they are not punished academically.

Today, other than Olympic participants, the athletes most likely to be tested for drugs are college athletes. Many doctors, coaches, trainers, school administrators, and drug experts think that urine testing for the presence of performance enhancing and/or recreational drugs is an essential part of athletic competition.[3]

Intent of Drug Testing

Drug testing in competitive sports was first implemented in the 1965 Tour of Britain Cycle Race and then used again in the 1968 Summer and Winter Olympic Games. It was designed to eliminate any competitive advantage that might result from the use of performance enhancing substances. Initially, drug testing was aimed at accomplishing the following goals:[4]

    1. Protect the health of the athletes

    2. Maintain the ethic of competition

    3. Maintain the quality of competition

As reports and concerns of recreational drug abuse rose, sports officials added other goals to the list:[5]

    1. Protect other athletes from injury caused by the drug abusing athlete

    2. Screen teams or groups of athletes for evidence of drug abuse

    3. Counsel and evaluate individuals identified as having a drug problem

    4. Enhance the role model perceptions of athletes

    5. Deter drug abuse by athletes

    6. Minimize criminality

URINE CONTROL AND CUSTODY FORM

Sample No. 060-11-498

SS Central Systems Labs., Ltd.
103 Henry Blvd. • Sedalia, MO 65301 • (816) 826-1779

TO BE COMPLETED BY DONOR

Name or Specimen Identification: **RONALD JOHNSON**
Employee ID # (SSN or Donor #): **488-42-5708**
Sex: **M**

Name or Specimen Identification:
Employer Name: **EUCLID College**

Medications in the past 15 days: **Tylenol, Clinoril, Sudafed**

I acknowledge that the specimen provided is my own and has not been altered in any way. I have verified that the number on the container and this form are identical. I hereby release this sample to the custody of the person signing below.

Signature: **Ronald Johnson** Date: **7/21/92**
Sample Received By: **Susan Merfeld** Date: **7/21/92**

PANEL

- [ ] Per Contract
- [x] Drugs of Abuse
- [ ] Drugs of Abuse (Extended Panel)
- [x] Anabolic Steroids
- [ ] Other: _____

"EXAMPLE"

REASON FOR TEST

- [ ] Preemployment
- [ ] Post Accident
- [ ] Random
- [x] Athletic
- [ ] Other (specify): _____

COLLECTION

Collector must note that temperature of specimen has been read. • Within Range • Temperature **96°**
Temp. indicator will change color if urine is within 90–100 F.

• Volume **3/4** • PH **6.0** • Sp. Gr. **1.019**

Comments:

I certify that the specimen identified on this form is the specimen presented to me by the donor, and that it has been collected, labeled and sealed as required by the instructions provided.

Collector's name (Please Print): **Suzan Merfeld**
X Signature of Collector: **Susan Merfeld**

Collection Facility and Location: **Arena - Training Room**
Telephone: **(216) 337-8681**
Client Company Name: **Athletic Dept.**

Adapted from Form 002738, American BioTest Laboratories, Inc.

Body Fluid to be Tested

Urine is the body fluid most frequently analyzed for evidence of illegal drug use by student athletes. The testing method is called urinalysis. A test is said to be positive if a predetermined amount of a banned substance is found in an athlete's urine.[6]

Several factors favor the testing of urine over other body fluids or tissues:[5]

> urine collection is not invasive
>
> large volumes can be collected easily
>
> drugs and their metabolites are generally present in higher concentrations in urine than in other fluids or tissues
>
> drugs and their metabolites are usually very stable in frozen urine, allowing for long-term storage

How Student Athletes are Tested?

Urine samples are collected under strictly controlled conditions. A testing official is assigned to each athlete to be tested and stays with the athlete throughout the testing procedure. Because offenders have devised many unique and ingenious ways of tampering with urine samples, a testing official must visibly witness the athlete voiding urine to ensure accurate test results. This visual inspection, though necessary, can be a source of stress and embarrassment for some student athletes. However, athletes who refuse to submit to testing are usually ruled ineligible to compete.

Most organizations divide each urine sample into two parts at the time of testing: samples A and B. To ensure confidentiality, the samples are assigned numbers for identification. The athlete is usually asked to label and seal the urine samples for mailing and storage in the presence of a testing official. The two samples are then sent to a certified testing laboratory.

At the testing laboratory, the final phases of drug testing are carried out. The procedure is performed in two steps. Step one, *Immunoassay*, is used to screen large numbers of urine samples and identify broad categories of drugs, except anabolic steroids. If the test identifies a drug in the urine sample, then step two is performed.[7]

Step two, *Gas Chromatography* with *Mass Spectroscopy*, not only confirms the presence of a drug in the urine but identifies the illegal substance.[8] The mass spectrometer uses an electron beam to explode the drug molecules into smaller pieces called molecular fingerprints and positively identifies the drug.[7]

To verify the positive test result, the procedure is repeated on the "B" sample of urine. If this sample is also positive, the athlete is notified and sanctions are enforced.

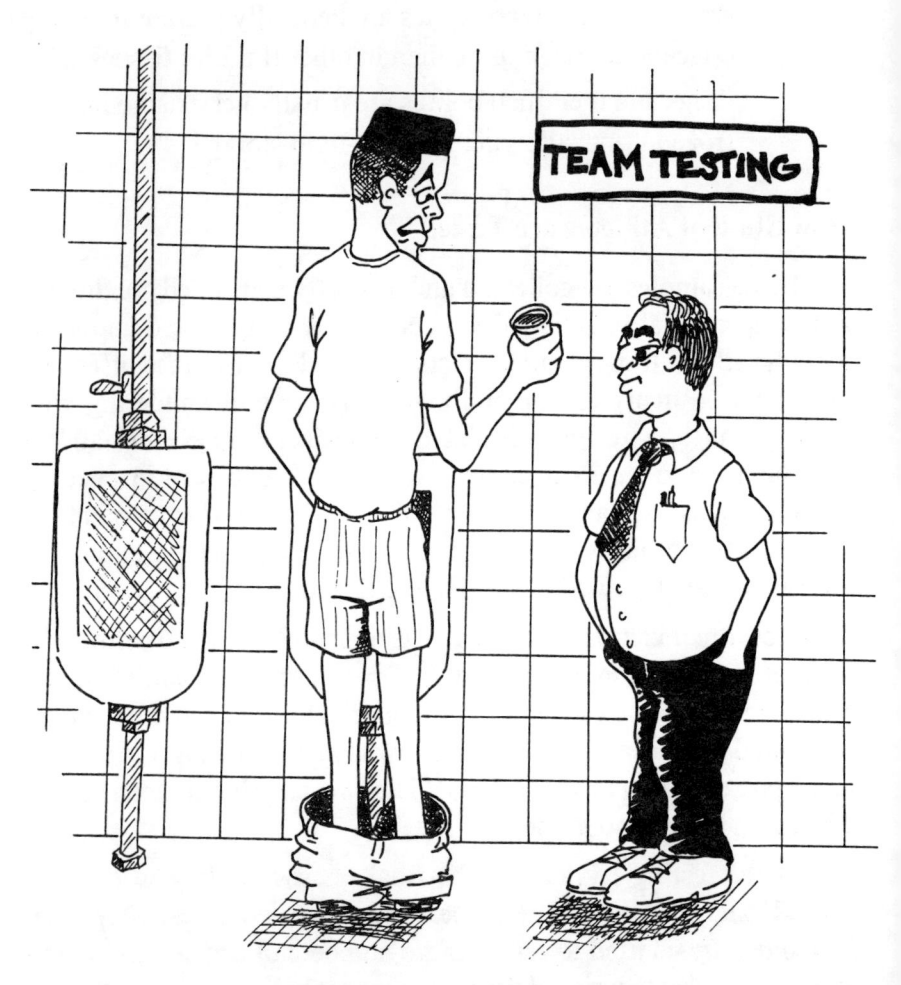

"You mean you have to watch?"

False Positives and False Negatives

Questions surrounding the reliability of drug testing surface almost as often as reports of positive tests. It isn't surprising then that denial of a positive urinalysis is a common response.

However, the technology used to identify a given chemical in the body is highly sophisticated. A certified International Olympic Committee (IOC) laboratory on the U.C.L.A. campus has performed "more than 18,000 tests and has never had a test result overturned."[9] Therefore, it's safe to say that if you test positive for a drug, the substance is likely to be in your body.

Although drug testing is nearly foolproof, two basic errors can occur. They are false positives and false negatives. A false positive occurs when an illicit drug is wrongly detected in an innocent person. A false negative identifies someone as innocent who has been using a banned substance.[8]

A false positive test result can be extremely damaging to you as a student athlete because your freedom, scholarship, reputation, and career may hinge on the test results. However, these results are so meticulously scrutinized and confirmed with the latest technology that there is little chance for a false positive to occur.[8]

False negatives, however, occur more frequently and generate the most concern when it comes to drug testing for student athletes. Anabolic steroids taken to enhance the student athlete's training efforts are difficult to detect since they are usually taken in the off-season and away from campus, long before competition begins. This time-lag between ingestion and competition gives the drugs ample time to be eliminated from the body. Therefore, the student athlete may test negative for a drug even though he or she is under the influence of a banned substance.

Banned substances such as stimulants and narcotics are taken to enhance performance during competition. They are easier to detect since they are taken such a short time prior to the event.

Questions that Positive Tests Fail to Answer

Despite sophisticated drug testing, a positive drug screen cannot answer some pertinent facts. These include the pattern and extent of drug use, the amount and exact time of use, the mode of administration (smoked, ingested, injected), and whether or not the user is addicted.

Hair Analysis to Determine Drug Use

The detection of some drugs by urinalysis is often limited by the short half-life of the drugs and their metabolites in the adult body. Cocaine, for example, cannot normally be detected in urine after one week to 10 days.

A relatively new and controversial method of drug testing has been introduced to counter the limitations of urinalysis. This technique analyzes human hair for the presence of drugs by means of radioimmunossay (RIA). This technique is primarily used to detect cocaine use. However, it can also be used to detect the use of marijuana, barbiturates, amphetamines, morphine, phencyclidine (PCP), methaqualone, and LSD.[10]

Hair grows approximately 1.0 to 1.5 centimeters a month. With this method it is possible to section the hair to show patterns of drug use, revealing long-term rather than recent exposure.[10]

Through hair analysis, student athletes who have negative urinalysis results and who deny drug use can still be identified since hair analysis reveals not only what drugs have been taken but when.[5] In this way hair analysis supplements rather than replaces urine testing.

Diuretics and Drug Testing

Diuretics are a class of drugs that are used in the treatment of hypertension and edema.[5] Athletes have traditionally used diuretics to assist in rapid weight loss. The drug's effects can benefit boxers and wrestlers since these athletes need to "make weight" quickly in order to qualify for a particular weight class.[11]

Some athletes take diuretics in an effort to avoid the detection of illegal substances in their bodies. Since diuretics increase urine formation and secretion, these athletes hope to eliminate the drug and thereby decrease the likelihood of testing positive for banned substances.[5,11]

To curtail this practice, the NCAA and the IOC include diuretics on their list of banned classes of drugs.[5] The USOC does not list diuretics as one of its banned substances. Caffeine and alcohol also act as diuretics, and all three organizations (NCAA, USOC, IOC) have banned these drugs but for reasons other than that they are diuretics.[11]

Sports Organizations That Test Student Athletes

National Collegiate Athletic Association (NCAA)
6201 College Boulevard
Overland Park, KS 66211-2422

United States Olympic Committee (USOC)
1750 E. Boulder St.
Colorado Springs, CO 80909-5760

The USOC primarily tests for drugs that can be used to enhance performance, while the NCAA tests not only for performance enhancers but also for street drugs.[6]

NCAA AND USOC DRUG TESTING FOR UNITED STATES ATHLETES

TESTING POLICY

NCAA
Member institutions

USOC
Provides a list of banned

are provided a list of banned substances; administers tests at NCAA championships and football games.

drugs to National Governing Bodies (NGBS); administers test at Olympic and Pan Am trials USOC sponsored competitions, and when requested, at NGB events.

BANNED DRUGS

NCAA
Psychomotor and CNS stimulants, anabolic steroids, "street drugs," diuretics, in some sports, alcohol and beta-blockers, and all tobacco products at championships.

USOC
Stimulants, narcotics analgesics, anabolic steroids, systemic corticosteroids, diuretics, and in some sports, beta-blockers, sedatives, hypnotics, tranquilizers, depressants, anti-convulsants, and alcohol.

WHO GETS TESTED

NCAA
Procedure to choose athletes to be tested are sports specific but may include random selection, position of finish, suspicion of use, playing time, and position.

USOC
Most top finishers at NGB and USOC sponsored competitions; a random sampling of other finishers and participants at training camps; all prospective team members at Olympic trials.

WHEN TEST ARE DONE

NCAA
Before, during, or after events, depending on institution and event; usually within 1 hour after an event.

USOC
Within 1 hour after event; frequency of tests varies with each NGB; alcohol may be tested before event.

PENALTY FOR POSITIVE TEST

NCAA
Athlete is deemed ineligible for post-season championship for minimum of 90 days; if retested positive, athlete will lose postseason eligibility for current season and succeeding season.

USOC
Athlete is suspended 6 months from USOC and NGB activities; repeat offenders suspended for 4 years; some NGBs have stiffer penalties.

NCAA Banned Drug Classes 1991-92[12]

Bylaw 31.2.3.1 Banned Drugs

(a) Psychomotor and Central Nervous System Stimulants:

amiphenazole	meclofenoxate
amphetamine	methamphetamine
bemigride	methylphenidate
benzphetamine	nikethamide
caffeine	norpseudoephedrine
chlorphentermine	pemoline
cocaine	pentetrazol
cropropamide	phendimetrazine
crothetamide	phenmetrazine
diethylpropion	phentermine
dimethylammphetamine	picrotoxine
doxapram	pipradol
ethamivan	prolintane
ethylamphetamine	strychnine
fencamfamine	And Related Compounds

(b) Anabolic steroids:

boldenone	nandrolone
clostebol	norethandrolone
dehydrochlomethyl-testosterone	oxandrolone
	fluoxymesterone
oxymesterone	mesterolone
oxymetholone	methenolone
stanozolol	methandienone
testosterone	methyltestosterone
And Related Compounds	

(c) Substances banned for specific sports:
Rifle:

alcohol	propranolol
atenolol	timolol
metoprolol	And Related
nadolol	Compounds
pindolol	

(d) Diuretics:

acetazolamide	hydroflumethiazide
bendroflumethiazide	methyclothiazide
benzhiazide	metolazone
bumetanide	polythiazide
chlorothiazide	quinethazone
chlorthalidone	spironolactone
ethacrynic acid	triamterene
flumethiazide	trichlormethiazide
furosemide	And Related

hydrochlorothiazide   Compounds

(e) Street Drugs:

heroin   **THC**
marijuana   **(tetrahydrocannabinol)**

(f) Definition of positive depends on the following:

for caffeine--if the concentration in urine exceeds 15 micrograms/ml.

for testosterone--if the administration of testosterone or the use of any other manipulation has the result of increasing the ratio of the total concentration of testosterone to that of epitestosterone in the urine to greater than 6:1.

for marijuana and THC--if the concentration in the urine of THC metabolite exceeds 25 nanogram/ml.

(From 1991-92 NCAA Drug Testing/Education Programs. NCAA Publishing 6201 College Boulevard Overland Park, Kansas 66211- 2422)

CONCLUSION

Seeking that elusive competitive edge, some athletes remain on the lookout for new, unorthodox, and even painful ways to avoid detection of illegal drug use. Some female athletes have inserted condoms filled with "clean" urine into their vaginas, then pierced the condoms with pins to release the urine into the collection containers.[13] At a Canadian Drug Inquiry, weight lifters Paramjit Gill, David Bolduc, and Raphael Zuffellato testified that they aquired "clean" urine from their coaches and "injected it into their bladders via catheters inserted up their penises" to mask their use of banned substances.[7]

Drug testing laboratories are working hard to keep pace with athletes who are continually learning about new resources and techniques to mask drug use. Even with the new sophisticated technology to detect illegal substance use, drug testing alone will not deter all student athletes from using drugs in an attempt to gain a competitive edge over their opponents. Dr. Andrew Pipe of the Sports Medicine Council of Canada nicely summarizes the problem, "Relying on drug testing to solve the problem of drug taking in sports is like relying on the Breathalyzer to solve the problem of drinking and driving."[14]

No, drug testing is not the cure-all to drug use in sports. However, coupled with education, drug testing is the most effective deterrent available to-date. Toward this end, most college and professional sports conferences and federations have now started random, unannounced drug testing. They hope that this dual approach will discourage the use of drugs, if not eliminate them from athletics.[8]

References

1. Schwartz RH: Urine Testing in the Detection of Drugs of Abuse. Arch Intern Med-Vik 148, November 1988.
2. N.C.A.A News: September 12, 1988.
3. Cowart VS: Medical News and PerspectiveS: Alcohol and Athletics Don't Mix, Can the Players Now learn to say "Nix?" JAMA, September 25, 1987-Vol 258, No.12.
4. Cowart VS: Medical News and Perspectives: Accord on Drug Testing, Sanctions Sought Before 1992 Olympics in Europe, JAMA, December 16, 1988-Vol 260, No. 23.
5. Wadler GI, Hainline B: Drugs and the Athlete. Philadelphia, F.A. Davis Company 1989.
6. Gall SL, et al: Who test which athletes for what drugs? The Physician and SportsMedicine, vol 16 No. 2, 1988.
7. Dealy Jr. FX: Win at any Cost. The Sell Out of College Athletics. 1990 Birch Lane Press Book, Carol Publishing Group.
8. Yesalis CE, Kammerer RC: The Strength and Frailities of Drug Tests. The New York Times, Sunday, February 4, 1990.
9. Cowart, p. 3398.
10. Graham K, Gideon K, et al: Determination of Gestional Cocaine Exposure by Hair Analysis. JAMA, December 15, 1989-Vol 262, N0. 23.
11. Williams MH: Beyond Training. How Athletes Enhance Performance Legally and Illegally. 1989 Leisure Press. Champaign, IL
12. 1991-92 NCAA Drug Testing/Education Programs. NCAA Publishing 6201 College Boulevard Overland Park, Kansas 66211-2422

13. Voy R: Drugs, Sports and Politics. Leisure Press 1991.
14. Cowart, p. 3398

Chapter 6

Human Growth Hormone
(hGH)

Although the use of human growth hormone (hGH) by athletes is a relatively new phenomenon, it is one more substance to add to the long history of athletes looking for something to give them a competitive edge on their opponents. Since little is known scientifically about hGH as a performance enhancer, its medical uses must be examined to understand the side effects.

What Is Human Growth Hormone?

HGH is not a steroid but a hormone produced by the pituitary gland and released in the body throughout life. Nearly all of the organs are dependent on hGH for proper growth and development.[1] It has been called the most powerful anabolic (tissue building) hormone known.[2] Adult males produce between 0.4 to 1.0 mg of hGH per day, while adolescents and females produce slightly more.

The effects of the hormone vary with an individual's age, sex, and stage of maturity. Severe deficiency of the hormone during childhood results in dwarfism.[3] Overproduction causes gigantism. Some children deficient in hGH have grown to normal adult height when treated with extracts of hGH.

Prior to 1985, hGH was obtained from cadaver pituitary extracts removed at the time of autopsy. Although distribution of hGH was tightly restricted, the hormone was available from the National

Hormone and Pituitary Program in Baltimore, Maryland.[3] After 1985, synthetic human growth hormone became commercially available.[1]

For many years athletes and body builders have been injecting human growth hormone in an attempt to increase muscle size and strength. Despite the lack of scientific studies validating hGH's effectiveness as a performance-enhancer, athletes continue to use the hormone. Competitors usually use hGH in conjunction with steroids but often quit using steroids and use the hormone alone before participating in athletic contests where they may be tested for drugs.[4]

Athletes and hGH

Athletes give the following reasons for using the hormone:
1. Increases muscle size
2. Reduces body fat
3. Cannot be detected by urinalysis
4. Does not pose health risks associated with anabolic steroids

How Much Does hGH Cost?

Although the use of hGH is steadily increasing, its prohibitive cost limits the abuse potential. The amount of hGH needed to elicit a performance-enhancing response costs around $1,000 for a two-month supply or somewhere between $6,000 and $10,000 a year.[5]

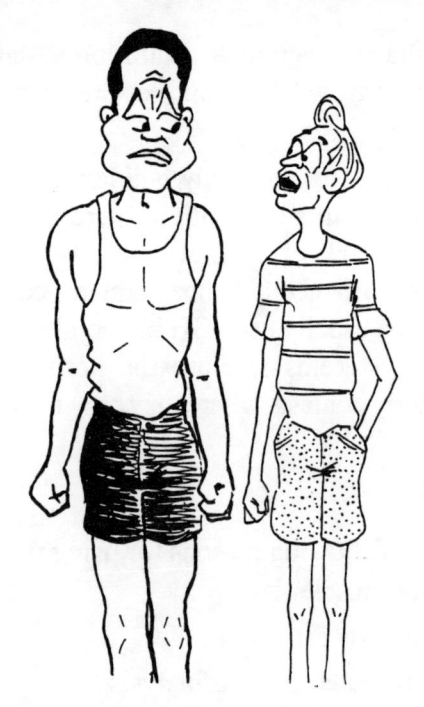

"You're not from around here are you?"

Negative Health Effects

As a student athlete, you need to be aware of the dangers associated with hGH abuse. The most common side effect of hGH is *acromegaly* . Acromegaly is the overgrowth of body organs, bones, and facial features. Height does not increase since the growth plates are already fused. Bones and connective tissue continue to grow, becoming so thick that sufferers can no longer wear rings or shoes. Facial features become grotesque due to the overgrowth of the brow bone, jaw, and soft tissue. The lungs and heart may double in size, and muscular weakness and joint laxity may develop.[4]

Other health problems associated with acromegaly include: [5]
1. Diabetes
2. Heart or thyroid disease
3. Menstrual disorders
4. Decreased sex drive

Animal Growth Hormone

Nonhuman growth hormone typically made from beef or pork glands (although occasionally extracts from monkeys are used), produces no physiological effect.[4]

Injecting animal growth hormone into the body can be very risky. Injected animal products may induce antibody formations that may neutralize the body's normal growth hormone.[4] Animal growth hormone is often fraudulently sold on the black market as human growth hormone.

A Risky Gamble

Parents who want to help their children gain more height and weight by using hGH need to be especially cautious about the possible adverse health effects of genuine hGH and about the existence of fraudulent products passing for hGH.

Because the hormone produces many irreversible, debilitating, and life threatening effects, using hGH in hopes of gaining performance enhancement is a very dangerous gamble.

References

1. Wadler GI, Hainline B: Drugs and the Athlete. Philadelphia, F.A. Davis Company 1989.
2. Taylor WN: Anabolic Steroids and the Athlete. McFarland and Company, Inc., 1982.
3. Council on Scientific Affairs: Drug Abuse in Athletes. Anabolic Steroids and Human Growth Hormone. JAMA, 259:11, March 18, 1988.
4. Strauss RH: Anabolic Steroids: Drugs and Performance In Sports. W.B. Saunders Company 1987.
5. Cowart VS: Human Growth Hormone: The Latest Ergogenic Aid? The Physician and SportsMedicine, vol 16 No. 3, March 1988.

Chapter 7
Blood Doping and Erythropoietin

BLOOD DOPING

Blood doping refers to the practice of intravenously infusing blood into the body in order to increase the amount of red blood cells and hemoglobin.[1] Since hemoglobin carries oxygen in the blood, blood doping increases the amount of oxygen that can be transported to the working muscle.[1] Increasing the oxygen content of arterial blood allows the athlete to obtain maximal aerobic power to improve his or her performance in endurance sports. This enhanced performance capacity has been shown to last from 2 to 18 days.[2]

What Sports Benefit From Blood Doping?

Blood doping is beneficial in sports that work the large muscle groups over prolonged periods of time.[2] The primary sports include long-distance running, cross-country skiing, and cycling

Blood doping has been shown to be effective in enhancing athletic performance. In controlled studies of well-trained athletes, blood doping increased aerobic endurance capacity from 10 percent to 25 percent.[1,2]

How Is Blood Doping Performed?

There are two methods of blood doping: homologous transfusion and autologous transfusion.[1] With the first method, you receive blood from another person whose blood is compatible with yours. Your normal red blood cell level is increased by the amount that is transfused.[3]

With the second method, some units of blood are removed from your own body a few weeks prior to an athletic event. The red blood cells are separated from the plasma, mixed with glycerol, and frozen. This process preserves the blood cells for an indefinite period of time. During the weeks prior to reinfusion, you retrain to full aerobic capacity, allowing the body to manufacture new red blood cells and return the red blood cell level to normal. About a week prior to the athletic event, the frozen red blood cells are thawed, reconstituted in a saline solution, and infused intravenously over a one or two hour period.[1,3]

Adverse Effects

When trained personnel perform blood tranfusions using approved techniques and store and label the blood in a registered blood bank, the procedure is usually safe. However, the use of donated blood poses several potential risks. These risks include: [1,3]

Immune Side Effects
    1. Fever
    2. Shock
    3. Chills
    4. Nausea
    5. Severe skin irritations

Viral Infections
    1. Hepatitis
    2. Liver infections
    3. Acquired immune deficiency syndrome (AIDS)

Using your own rather than donated blood also carries certain risks. A flaw in technique can lead to complications such as bacterial infections. Human error might allow air to be injected into the blood stream that could cause a fatal heart attack. The greatest risk involves mislabeling blood. Receiving a transfusion of the wrong blood type could be fatal.

Legal Rights and Privileges

Blood doping has been banned by the National Collegiate Athletic Association (NCAA), the United States Olympic Committee (USOC), and the International Olympic committee (IOC). The American College of Sports Medicine views blood doping by student athletes as unethical.[3]

Evidence confirming blood doping can lead to punitive actions by the NCAA and the other athletic-governing bodies.

ERYTHROPOIETIN

Erythropoietin (EPO) is a hormone produced by the kidneys that stimulates the production of red blood cells.[1] If the kidneys are damaged, the EPO level drops and you become anemic. Regular blood transfusions are then necessary.[4] Through the process of biotechnology, researchers looking for ways to increase the blood supplies of surgery patients or those suffering from kidney failure have developed a method of producing EPO in the laboratory.[5] The recombinant erythropoietin is virtually identical to the naturally occurring hormone.[4]

Medical Uses

Approved by the Food and Drug Administration (FDA) in June 1989, EPO has many legitimate therapeutic uses. EPO has been hailed as a wonder drug since it allows patients awaiting surgery to increase the amount of blood they can store and use. It has been approved to treat anemia caused by chemotherapy or the AIDS drug, AZT, and it is projected to aid in the treatment of cancer, leukemia, and arthritis.[5]

Since its approval, EPO has become a huge marketing success. Amgen, the company with exclusive rights in the United States sold $304.2 million of the drug in 1991.[6]

Effects on Performance

EPO boosts your body's production of red blood cells and thereby increases the amount of oxygen carried throughout the body. Theoretically it should also improve athletic performance. Since athletes often look for ways to increase their chances in competition, it didn't take them long to recognize the possible performance enhancing benefits of EPO and seek it out for use.

A study of 15 Swedish athletes conducted by the Stockholm Institute of Gymnastics and Sports concluded that EPO does in fact enhance athletic performance. The test results showed an improvement of nearly 10 percent in aerobic exercise after use of the drug.[6]

Bjorn Ekblom, the Swedish exercise physiologist who pioneered blood doping, tested top Swedish athletes with EPO and concluded in an unpublished report that the drug could cut 30 seconds off a 20 minute racing time. However, questions have been raised regarding testing methods and reliability of Ekblom's results.[4]

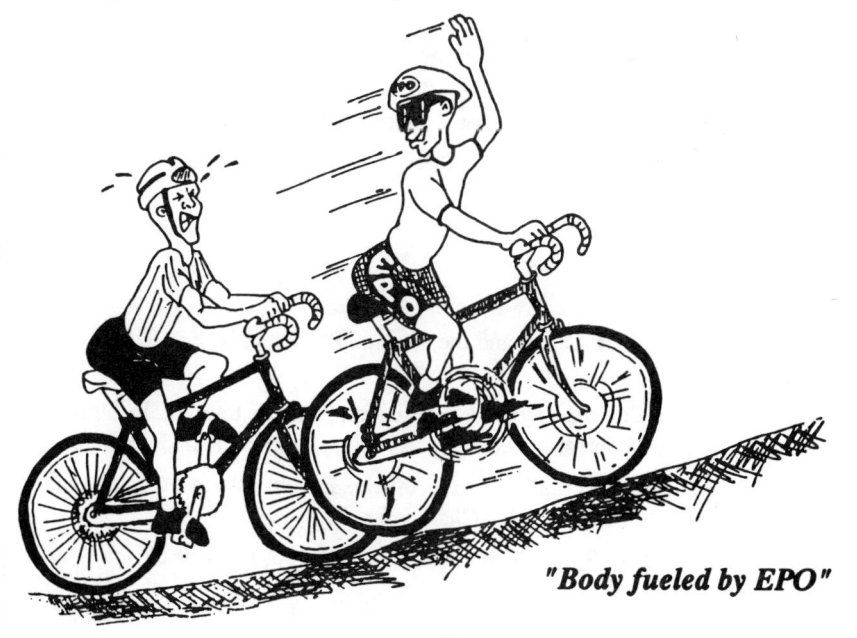

"Body fueled by EPO"

Adverse Effects

Although EPO may excite many athletes looking for a competitive advantage, it is important to know that use of the drug brings with it some potentially deadly side effects.

Taking EPO to boost your red blood cell count causes the blood to thicken, and the normal dehydration that occurs in competition causes the blood to thicken even more. The thicker your blood, the greater your chances are for many life threatening health problems such as hypertension, blood clots, strokes, and heart attacks.[4,5]

Between 1987 and 1990, as many as 17 European professional cyclists "mysteriously" died. Doctors working with the athletes reported the cause of death as, "some kind of heart failure."[7] Although the doctors denied any knowledge of EPO use by the cyclists, some sports medicine and blood specialists suspect the deaths were linked to use or abuse of the drug.[4,5] No deaths have been reported in sports other than cycling. Other aerobic endurance athletes such as marathon runners and cross-country skiers have also been suspected of using the drug; however, no complications have been reported.[6]

The use of laboratory produced erythropoietin (EPO) is considered safe and effective when properly used in medical treatment. However, to use the drug for performance enhancement, is like playing with a loaded gun. Deadly consequences are always a risk. Yes, EPO can increase your aerobic capacity, but it can also kill you. When considering whether or not to use this dangerous drug, each student athlete must ask him or herself, "Just what price am I willing to pay for the all mighty W?"

References

1. Wadler GI, Hainline B: Drugs and the Athlete. Philadelphia, F.A. Davis Company 1989.
2. Ekblom B: Blood doping, oxygen breathing, and altitude training. In Strauss, RH (ed): Drugs and Performance In Sports. WB Saunders, Philadelphia, 1987.
3. Williams MH: Beyond Training: How Athletes Enhance Performance Legally and Illegally. 1989 Leisure Press. Champaign, IL.
4. Kim A: A Bad Boost. Sports Illustrated, November 26, 1990. p. 29

5. Jereski L: It Gives Athletes A Boost--Maybe Too Much. Business Week, December 11, 1989.
6. Fisher LM: Stamina-Building Drug Linked to Athlete's Deaths. New York Times, May 19, 1991 Section 1 pg. 22.
7. Kim, p. 29

Chapter 8
Stimulants

A *stimulant* is any drug that increases alertness and energy, reduces hunger, and provides a feeling of well-being.[1] From a medical standpoint, stimulants are "agents that help to increase functional ability."[2]

In the world of athletics, stimulants are among the most popularly used and abused performance-enhancing drugs. They are easily obtained and readily used in mainstream society. Hardly a day goes by that these drugs are not consumed by most student athletes in one form or another.

Why Do Student Athletes Take Stimulants?

The use of stimulants in the student athlete population is widespread due to their ability to "mask, delay, or alter the perception of fatigue."[3] Generally, when student athletes take stimulants for other than medical reasons they do so with the intent of delaying fatigue, controlling weight, or gaining a performance advantage over their opponents. *Amphetamines, cocaine, nicotine, ephedrine* (in nasal decongestants) and *caffeine* are commonly used stimulants.[4,2]

CAFFEINE

Because of its ability to elevate mood, mask fatigue, and increase wakefulness, caffeine is popular within all segments of society. In recent years caffeine has gained in popularity among athletes, especially among long distance runners and cyclists, because it delays the onset of fatigue, resulting in more productivity and faster times. [2,4]

No doubt you already know that since caffeine is a drug, there is no way to guarantee a consistent effect for all users. It is equally impossible to guarantee the same effect each time for the same user.[3] You probably also realize that heavy caffeine consumption is not without consequences. Psychological or physiological dependence may ensue. Heavy users experience withdrawal symptoms when they stop consuming the product. The following symptoms are common:[5]

>fatigue
>
>irritability
>
>headaches
>
>decreased concentration
>
>depression

Caffeine's popularity, legal standing, and conflicting research studies on effectiveness and dosage have kept it from being banned altogether by the athletic governing bodies. However, the consumption of high doses of caffeine (greater than 10 micrograms per ml.) is considered to be illegal in most sporting events due to the drug's potential performance-enhancing effects. The International Olympic Committee (IOC) defines *caffeine doping* as greater than 12 micrograms per ml of caffeine in the urine. The NCAA urine limit for caffeine is 15 micrograms per ml.

According to some estimates, 2 cups of coffee will produce urine levels of 3 to 6 micrograms per ml.[4] According to this standard, 5 to 6 cups of brewed coffee one hour prior to competition will produce enough caffeine in the urine to fail a drug test.

Caffeine can be found in the following sources:[2]
coffee
cola soda
coco
tea
chocolate
aspirin

NICOTINE

Drugs and the Athlete[6]

On February 25, 1984, a young, talented, grit-tough, Oklahoma high school senior looked up from his bed, smiled, and gave a "thumbs up" sign to his sister. A short time later, he died.

Sean Marsee, an eighteen-year old student athlete, had always been a stickler for home, school, and team rules. He was the oldest of five children raised in a single parent home and provided a positive role model for his younger siblings. Sean, a consummate team player, was disciplined and caring, and had always kept himself in perfect mental and physical condition. Sean lifted weights, watched his diet, ran five miles a day, and didn't drink or smoke. At five-foot-five, 130 pounds, the Talihina High School star athlete had won 28 track medals as an anchor for the 400-meter relay team.

Sean Marsee had one habit however, since the age of twelve he had been using smokeless tobacco. He briefly used chewing tobacco but soon started dipping snuff. Shortly thereafter, enjoying the nicotine rush, Sean was "never without a dip." [7] *Always conscious of his appearance, Sean swallowed the snuff rather than be seen spitting in public.*

His mother, a registered nurse, warned Sean of the dangers associated with smokeless tobacco and valiantly tried to get him to stop. Since smoking and drinking were prohibited, Sean and many of his peers dipped to avoid breaking the training rules. His coach knew some of the guys were using chew and snuff but didn't think the problem was serious enough to stop them. Sean saw professional athletes selling snuff on television and didn't think it would be harmful to him. He had been using one can of snuff every day and a half.

At eighteen, Sean's attitude about snuff changed drastically when he noticed a large red sore with a hard white core on his tongue. The throat specialist who examined him described Sean's throat as one that appeared to belong to a 75-year old who had been dipping snuff for 72 years. After a positive biopsy in May 1983, Sean underwent surgery to remove part of his tongue. He was scheduled to undergo radiation therapy but before he had started, the doctor discovered that the cancer had spread to the nearby tissue and that additional surgery would be needed.

Approximately one month after his first surgery, Sean underwent an eight hour procedure to remove all lymph nodes, muscles, and blood vessels on the right side of his face. Five months later in November, a third surgery was required to remove the lower right jaw.

Sean went home from the hospital for Christmas. He kept his faith, maintained a positive attitude, and insisted on caring for himself as much as possible. Despite all the suffering, Sean still had thoughts and cravings for snuff. In January 1984, several lumps were found in the left side of his neck. The biopsy results were positive.

Sean Marsee remained emotionally strong during the final weeks of his life. He maintained his award winning "finishing kick" to the end. Six years after first starting to use smokeless tobacco, Sean Marsee was dead.

(Adapted from Fincher J: Sean Marsee's Smokeless Death. Readers Digest October 1985 p. 107-112.[6])

Nicotine, the drug in tobacco that causes addiction, has been referred to as the "most poisonous substance known to man."[5] This commonly abused stimulant has very little therapeutic value.

For years student athletes have used cigarettes and smokeless tobacco in hopes of getting a calming, stimulating, or performance-enhancing effect during competition. For example, reports in Texas indicate that one-third of the varsity football and baseball players regularly chew smokeless tobacco.[3] To my knowledge there is no research to support the claims that nicotine enhances athletic performance. It does not improve reaction time, movement time, or total response time.[2]

The two main types of smokeless tobacco, *chewing tobacco* and *snuff*, are marketed in several forms:

    1. *Compressed tobacco* is twisted into a block form, plug, or twist. The user breaks or bites off a piece and places it in the mouth between the lip or cheek and the lower gum.[4,8]

    2. *Loose leaf tobacco*, usually referred to as "chew," consists of strips or shreds sold in foil pouches. A golfball sized portion is placed between the cheek and gum where it is slowly sucked and chewed.[4,7]

    3. *Moist or dry powdered tobacco or "snuff"* is typically sold in small round cans, but it is also sold in small packets that look like tea bags. Dry snuff is a finely powdered tobacco placed in the nostrils. The more popular form of snuff is the moist type. The user takes a pinch and leaves it between the cheek or lip and gum. This practice is referred to as "dipping."[4,7]

Tobacco is often mixed with sugar and licorice to increase its appeal. Snuff is likely to be treated with flavors like wintergreen, mint, or menthol for the same reason.[7] Chewing tobacco and snuff were popular in the United States at the turn of the century, but the invention of the cigarette-rolling machine along with the high incidence of tuberculosis led to their replacement by smoking tobacco. Today, however, health concerns over smoking tobacco have led to the resurgence of smokeless tobacco use.[4]

In professional sports, smokeless tobacco became popular in the 1950s and flourished in the 1970s and 80s. It is still popular today.[4,9] In the 1970s, typical smokeless tobacco users were males over age 50. Today, most users are young males between ages 16 and 29. However, children as young as 8 or 9 are known to use smokeless tobacco.[7]

Despite the documented health hazards associated with the use of smokeless tobacco, many student athletes and coaches continue to use the products. Some users justify their habit by saying that it is safer than smoking cigarettes. This is erroneous, however, since smokeless tobacco is associated with higher risks for several types of cancer. Smokeless tobacco is also associated with an increase in stained teeth, tooth cavities, gum recession, and leukoplakia (white patches in the mouth).[10]

It seems to me that most smoking and smokeless tobacco use can be attributed to the aggressive and successful advertising campaigns of tobacco companies. For example, Benson and Hedges sponsors golf tournaments; Virginia Slims sponsors the women's tennis circuit; and the United States Tobacco Company, the manufacturer of snuff, spent over $1 million as an official sponsor of the 1980 Olympic Games.[4]

The rocky marriage between tobacco products and sports was seemingly consummated after cigarette ads were banned from the airwaves in 1971. As an alternative form of advertising, tobacco companies began posting logos and banners in the background of televised sports events. RJR Nabisco Inc, makers of Winston cigarettes, sponsors approximately 2,500 sporting events each year. It is estimated that the tobacco industry spends approximately $300 million annually on sports promotions and advertising.[11]

The following athletic events are also underwritten or sponsored by tobacco companies: [10]

Marlboro Challenge skiing

Winston Cup auto racing

Vantage Cup senior golf tour

Lucky Strike darts tournament

Winston Team America soccer series

Camel Motocross races

Benson & Hedges on Ice

Salem Pro-Sail races

Lucky Strike bowling.

The tobacco companies have been particularly successful in getting top professional athletes to advertise and glamorize their products.[4] Since sports superstars serve as highly visible role models, their advertising of tobacco products sends double messages and can produce credibility problems for other athletes and athletics.

Physical Effects

Few scientists or medical professionals doubt that nicotine adversely effects physical skills and athletic performances or causes major health problems. Every form of tobacco is physically addictive, and trying to stop automatically causes an intense craving for more.

Nicotine constricts the blood vessels which makes the heart work harder to pump blood throughout the body. Approximately thirty minutes after a cigarette is inhaled, the coronary arteries shrink 38 percent.[12] The chronic use of tobacco products lowers your resistance to diseases and decreases sperm production and testosterone levels.[13] Other negative physical effects are also associated with smoking and smokeless tobacco use:[5]

- heart disease
- impotence
- strokes
- gastrointestinal ailments
- lung, mouth, stomach, and throat cancer

For years the use of snuff has been ominously connected with oral cancer. Oral cancer ranks as one of the nation's top ten leading causes of cancer death. Research has shown that using snuff can produce high levels of *nitrosamines*. These cancer causing compounds are formed by the chemical interaction of saliva and tobacco in the mouth.[6] One dip of snuff produces as much nicotine as a cigar, but ten times the amount of nitrosamines.[6]

Secondary smoke inhalation poses significant health risks for the non-smoker. According to the United States Health and Human Services, smoke inhaled by the person smoking a cigarette contains

11.8 mg. of tar and .8 mg. of nicotine. Smoke inhaled by persons in close proximity to the smoker (passive inhalation) contains 22.1 mg. of tar and 1.4 mg. of nicotine.[5] Passive smoking also increases the risk of colds and pneumonia, sinusitis, and eczema and skin infections.[14]

Mental Effects

Regular users of nicotine who try to give up the habit can expect to experience the following withdrawal symptoms:[5]

tobacco cravings

sleep disturbances

tremors

irritability

decreased blood pressure and pulse rate

intellectual impairment

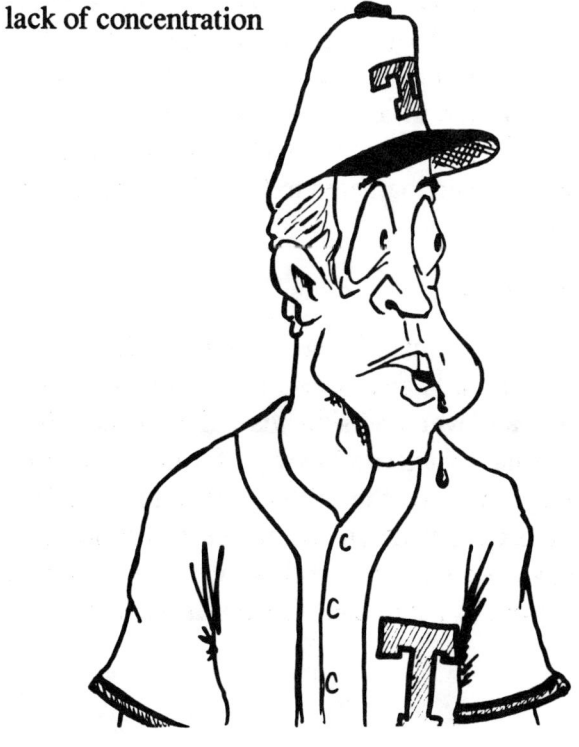

compulsive overeating

lack of concentration

School/Team Rules

Many schools or teams have policies that prohibit the use of tobacco products, usually smoking tobacco, by student athletes. Due to the known dangers associated with the consumption of nicotine, these rules are put in place to safe-guard your health. Paradoxically, these same rules are sometimes enforced by coaches, administrators, or others who smoke or chew themselves. While on the surface this behavior appears to be a clear double standard, a closer look reveals individuals who are caught up in a vicious habit that is extremely difficult to break: *nicotine addiction.* Staff members assigned to enforce the rules are usually painfully aware that they are sending double messages but they, like most users of tobacco products, are unable to stop. Eighty percent of all adult smokers wish they could quit.

EPHEDRINE

Ephedrine is a drug that stimulates the central nervous system. Available over-the-counter without a prescription, it is often combined with caffeine to mimic the action of amphetamines.[4] For this reason it is often referred to as a "look-alike drug." This practice began in the 1970s when ephedrine as well as may other psychoctive drugs were formulated and marketed to look like amphetamines.

Effects On Performance

Today ephedrine is primarily used as a nasal decongestant. An effective cold remedy, it is also useful in the treatment of asthma, allergic reactions, hay fever, and sinusitis. There is no reliable data to show that ephedrine enhances athletic performance. However, the drug is banned by some of the athletic governing bodies (IOC, USOC) because it is classified as a central nervous system stimulant. The NCAA removed ephedrine and other over the-counter-cold and diet medications from its list of banned substances in 1990.

Table 8.1
Banned Over-The-Counter Cold Medicines For Colds And Sinus Infections[2]

Ephedrine	Phenylephrine
Propylhexedrine	Pseudoephedrine
Phenylpropanolamine and related cold products	

American swimmer Rick DeMont was disqualified during the 1972 Olympic Games for taking medication containing ephedrine. Rick had been diagnosed as having asthma and reportedly was taking the drug for his condition. Despite appeals, the disqualification was upheld [4]

Table 8.2
Physical Effects

Some Physical Complications Associated with Ephedrine Use:

headaches	dizziness
heart palpitations	hypertension
anorexia	

Table 8.3
Mental Effects

Some Mental Complications Associated With Ephedrine Use:

agitation	confusion
nervousness	paranoia
hallucinations	

AMPHETAMINES

The most commonly abused stimulants by student athletes are *amphetamines*.

Amphetamines go by many street names:

Black Beauties	Speed
Ice	White Crosses
Crank	Uppers
Greenies	Dexies
Pep Pills	Crystal

Medical Uses

Amphetamines are prescribed for the following medical disorders:[3,2,4]

1. Cardiovascular complications
2. Obesity
3. Attention deficit disorders
4. Sleep disorders (narcolepsy)
5. Minimal brain dysfunction (hyperkinesis)
6. Colds and allergies
7. Asthma

Physical Effects

Research studies on amphetamines have revealed the following performance-enhancing effects:[3,2,4]

1. Increased blood flow from the heart
2. Improved endurance capacity
3. Improved aerobic endurance performance
4. Increased alertness
5. Increased concentration
6. Improved reaction time in fatigued persons

Amphetamines principally effect the central nervous system. Potential benefits derived from their use must be carefully weighed against the known negative side effects of the drugs.[4]

Strong stimulants such as amphetamines are not recommended for student athletes due to the high probability of medical complications.[2] Furthermore, abuse of these drugs can easily lead to drug addiction and overdose. "Convulsions, coma and death may follow severe central nervous system stimulation from amphetamine use."[4][15]

Table 8.4

The Negative Side Effects of Amphetamines include: [2][3]

Body water loss

Frequent urination

Increased heart rate

Increased blood pressure

Restricted blood flow to the skin

Abnormally high body temperature

These side effects can also raise the body temperature to dangerous levels, leading to serious heat illness such as heatstroke. [2]

Table 8.5

Amphetamine use is also responsible for the following ailments:[4]

Tremors	Nausea
Dizziness	Vomiting
Anorexia	Heart Palpitations

Amphetamines are used and abused by student athletes as a form of weight control due to their ability to suppress the appetite. As a result, eating disorders have increasingly been diagnosed in certain competitive activities such as gymnastics, swimming, ballet, wrestling, thoroughbred racing and women's tennis. These sports have the following features in common: they are individualized activities, they are entered into at a high level during the teenage years, and weight control is important. [4]

Mental Effects

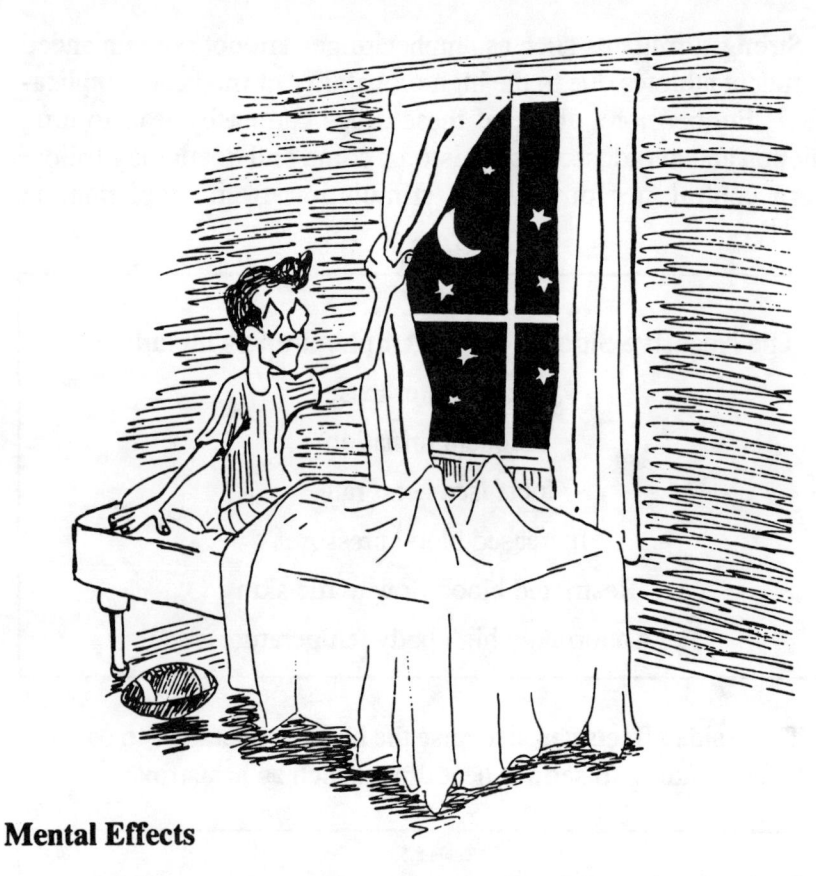

Amphetamines can cause a drowsy or exhausted person to feel more alert.[3] This occurs in part because stimulants, especially amphetamines and caffeine, increase excitability, arousal, and motivation.

The drugs produce other psychological effects as well:[4]
1. Elevation of mood
2. Increased initiative and self-confidence
3. Increased motor and speech activity

Amphetamines can overstimulate your central nervous system and cause you to become hyperactive, irritable, paranoid, and hypertalkative. They can also negatively effect decision making.

Effects On Performance

Extensive research on amphetamines shows that the positive physical response elicited in a body at rest does not necessarily transfer to a body that is exercising. It appears that the body's natural release of epinephrine (adrenaline) and other hormones during peak exercise overrides the effects of oral amphetamines. Heart rate, lung ventilation, blood flow, and oxygen intake therefore are not improved.[2]

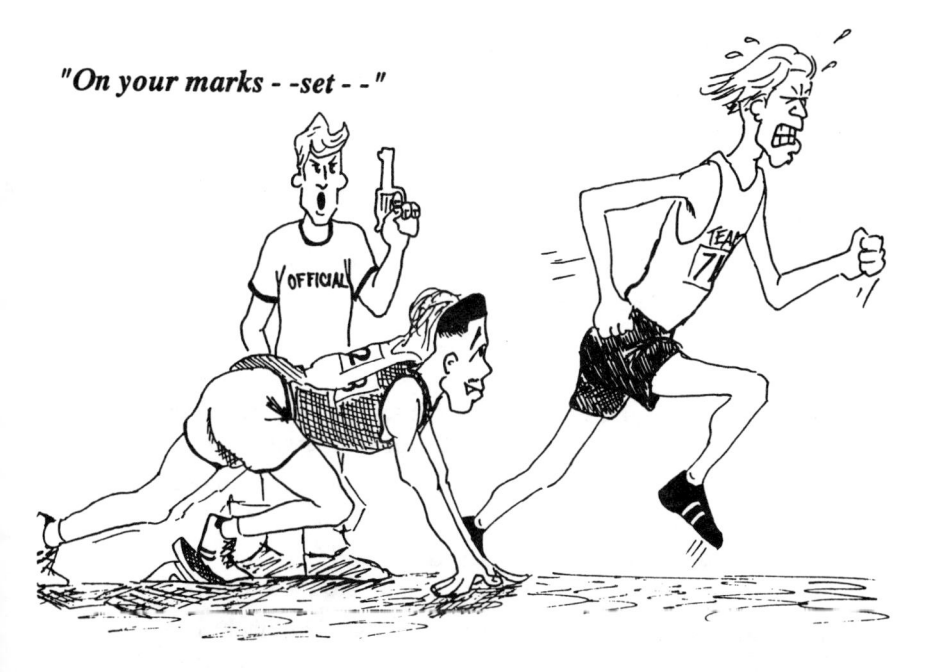

"On your marks - -set - -"

Legal Rights and Privileges

Most stimulants are banned by the governing sports bodies and are therefore illegal for student athletes to use. Stimulant drugs can be detected by all standard drug testing methods.

It is important for you to know that many over-the-counter medicines normally taken for colds, allergies, headaches, and other ailments contain stimulants that are banned for athletic competition. Sudafed, pseudoephedrine, Sinex, Nyquil, and Dristan are just a few. Therefore, great care should be exercised before treating everyday ailments with medication.

Banned drugs, even though prescribed by your doctor, are still banned drugs. If you will be competing in an athletic event where drug testing will be performed, you should check with your team doctor, coach, trainer, or athletic governing body about the legality of any medications you are taking.[2]

References

1. Sloan IJ: Alcohol And Drug Abuse And The Law. 1980 Oceana Publications, Inc.
2. Williams MH: Beyond Training: How Athletes Enhance Performance Legally and Illegally. 1989 Leisure Press. Champaign, IL
3. Lombardo JA: Stimulants. In Strauss, RH (ed): Drugs and Performance In Sports. WB Saunders, Philadelphia, 1987.
4. Wadler GI, Hainline B: Drugs and the Athlete. Philadelphia, F.A. Davis Company 1989.
5. Taylor P: Substance Abuse. 1988 Charles C. Thomas, Publisher
6. Fincher J: Sean Marsee's Smokeless Death. Readers Digest October 1985 p. 107-112.
7. Fincher, p. 107.
8. Squier CA: The Nature of Smokeless Tobacco and Patterns of Use. CA-A Cancer Journal For Clinicians. Vol. 38. No. 4 July/August 1988.
9. Glover E, et al: Implications Of Smokeless Tobacco Use Among Athletes. The Physician and SportsMedicine, vol 14 No. 12, March 1986.
10. Riley WT, Barenie JT, Myers DR: Typology and Correlates of Smokeless Tobacco Use. Journal Of Adolescent Health Care 1989; 10:357-362
11. Wichmann SA, Martin DR: Sports and Tobacco, The Smoke Has Yet to Clear. The Physician and SportsMedicine, vol 19 No. 11 November 1991.
12. Quillen: The New York Times. March 7, 1991 p. B 10.
13. Surgeon Generals Report. 1980
14. Journal of Can. Med. Assoc. 94: 1165-1171, 1966.
15. Wadler, p 84.

Chapter 9
Depressants

Depressants, in contrast to stimulants, sedate the central nervous system and decrease physiological functioning.[1] As a result, depressants are regularly used as sleep inducers, anxiety reducers, or relaxants.[2]

Barbiturates (typically used as sleeping aids) and *benzodiazepines* (often prescribed as muscle relaxants) are commonly known depressant drugs. However, the following drugs can also be classified as depressants because they produce calming, hypnotic, and sedative effects:

alcohol

morphine

marijuana

tranquilizers

Depressants are some of the most frequently prescribed and abused drugs in the United States. Their popularity is steady; they regularly account for a higher percentage of annual sales than birth control pills and penicillin.[3] Of all the prescribed depressant drugs, *Valium*, a benzodiazepine, ranks in the top ten.

A common slang name for depressants is *downers*. Other street names include: Barbs, Reds, Yellows, Christmas Trees, Blues, Devils, Yellow Jackets, purple Hearts, and Goofballs. However, *downers* is the name most often used when referring to this class of drugs.[3]

Effects on Performance

Like alcohol and marijuana, depressants are not generally known as performance-enhancing drugs. Many student athletes have asked me why anyone interested in higher performance would voluntarily take something that is known to restrict and even impair physical functioning.

There are several answers regarding this point. One reason might be that depressants slow down the central nervous system and in turn reduce the nervousness, muscle tremors, and anxiety that comes with competition. This slow down or sedating effect can benefit gymnasts, figure skaters, ski jumpers, and ballet dancers, since these performances suffer if the athlete is overly excited.[1] Sports which require hand steadiness such as rifle shooting, pistol shooting, and archery also require the athlete to be calm and relaxed.

Student athletes give the following reasons for using depressants:[1]

> to build confidence
>
> to increase the tolerance for pain
>
> to reduce daily stress which may affect performance

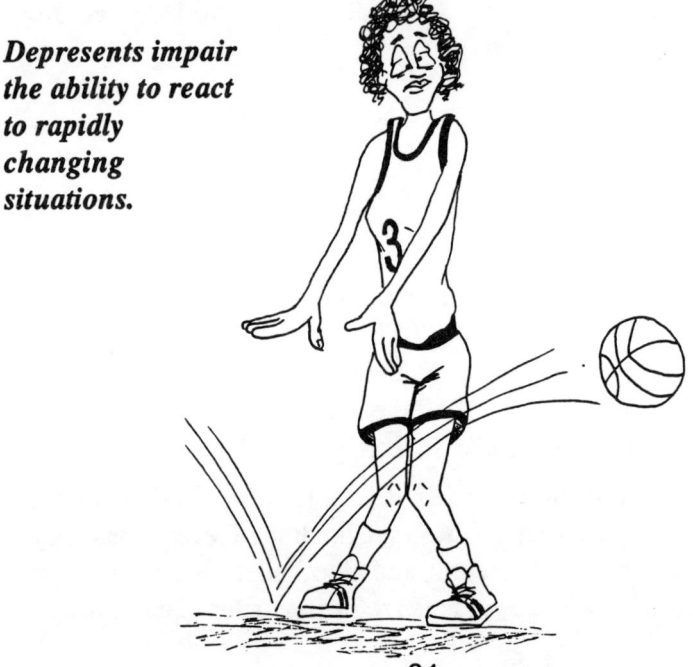

Depresents impair the ability to react to rapidly changing situations.

Physical and Mental Effects

Even though depressants have been shown to temporarily benefit some competitors, it must be emphasized that the drugs also have many negative side effects. They can produce physical as well as psychological dependence, and when abused, they can be fatal.

Depressants impair reaction time, visual tracking skills, and cognitive functioning. Countless research studies conclusively show that depressant drugs adversely affect athletic performance. The ability to make quick decisions and to react to rapidly changing situations is grossly impaired. [1]

Short term side effects of depressants include:[4]
- drowsiness
- sedation
- blurred vision
- slurred speech
- decreased attention span
- decreased memory
- impaired gait/balance

Long term or chronic effects of depressants include:[3]
- damage to the liver and pancreas
- deterioration of the central nervous system
- reduced sex drive
- convulsions
- hallucinations
- depression

Overdose of depressants has always been a problem. It is important to realize that the overdose potential rises significantly when the drugs are combined with alcohol. Small non-intoxicating amounts of alcohol, 1 or 2 ounces, mixed with 1 or 2 barbiturates or benzodiazepines may produce disastrous results. Overdose with depressants is further complicated by the fact that it is almost impossible to predict overdose levels when the drugs are mixed with alcohol.[5]

Most depressants are banned by the International Olympic Committee (IOC) due to their ability to reduce or mask pain. The student athlete's motivation and desire to compete and succeed is very strong. The possibility of severe or permanent injury to athletes who, with the help of pain killers, continue to compete was a major factor in the decision to ban the drugs.[1]

Summary

There are many dangers associated with depressant use. The greatest danger is death, although overdose and addiction are major concerns as well. Depressants do temporarily mask or alleviate the symptoms of tension and stress, but they are not necessary. Through the process of daily living you have developed coping mechanisms that will help you manage the unpleasant occurrences and uncertainties of competition, academics, and day to day life as a person and as a student athlete.

The use of depressants to sedate or numb you may lead you to neglect these coping skills. In turn you may come to depend on the drugs more and more to calm fears, anxieties, and insecurities. When this transition takes place, physical and psychological dependence is not far away.

References

1. Williams MH: Beyond Training: How Athletes Enhance Performance Legally and Illegally. 1989 Leisure Press. Champaign, IL
2. Lombardo JA: Stimulants. In Strauss, RH (ed): Drugs and Performance InSports. WB Saunders, Philadelphia, 1987.
3. Parker J: Downers: The Distressing Facts About Depressant Drugs. Do It Now Foundation (DIN) Phoeniz AZ February 1986.
4. Wadler GI, Hainline B: Drugs and the Athlete. Philadelphia, F.A. Davis Company 1989.
5. Parker J: Valium, Librium, and the Benzodiazepine Blues. Do It Now Foundation (DIN) Phoeniz AZ October 1985.

Chapter 10
Reasons, Explanations, Excuses.

Drugs and the Athlete

Hundreds of tragic stories highlight talented student athletes who "shoulda, woulda, or coulda" made it big in college or professional sports but fell prey to the seductions of alcohol and other drugs. None, however, compare to the tragedy still being played out of Lloyd Daniels.

Affectionately known as "Sweet Pea" due to his resemblance to the baby in the Popeye cartoons, Lloyd Daniels was touted to be as assured of success in basketball as the presence of sliced bread in the American household. Daniels, a 6' 8" forward, was hailed as the best high school basketball talent to come off the streets of New York City since Lew Alcindor (Kareem Abdul-Jabbar). He was said to be comparable to Magic Johnson in talent but with a better outside shot.[1] *By most accounts Lloyd Daniels, the playground legend, was certain to be an N.B.A. star.*

Lloyd Daniels grew up in rough New York neighborhoods. His mother died of cancer when he was three years old. His father, devastated by her death, left Sweet Pea to be raised by his grandmother who already had 11 children. Ultimately reared by both his maternal and paternal grandmothers, the youngster alternated be-

tween their homes in St. Albans, Queens, and the East New York section of Brooklyn.[3] Daniels grew up fast in this rough and unstable environment. Introduced to drugs at an early age, he was smoking marijuana by the time he was 10 years old.[2]

Lloyd Daniel's formal education was, for all intents and purposes, non-existent. According to his high school coaches, he frequently skipped classes. He attended four high schools in three states without ever receiving a diploma.[5] Daniels quit high school altogether in 1986 as a junior. He admitted to having poor reading skills (third grade level) and claimed that he didn't attend classes regularly because he didn't have too.[2] He was mercilessly and systematically passed through school because of his basketball skills. When he dropped out of Andrew Jackson High School in February 1986, Daniels was averaging 31.2 points, 12.3 rebounds, and 10 assists per game. He said he quit because he just didn't want to go anymore.[3]

Despite a lack of formal education, Daniels signed a letter of intent to play basketball for the University of Nevada-Las Vegas (UNLV) and was quickly enrolled for a semester at Mount San Antonio Junior College in Walnut, California. In 1987 he registered as a student at the UNLV campus, intending to play basketball for the premier college basketball power.[2,3]

Lloyd Daniels never played a game for the Runnin' Rebels; in fact he never even practiced with the team. In February 1987 Sweet Pea was busted in a Las Vegas crack house and charged with intent to buy cocaine from an undercover officer.[3] He was kicked off the basketball team, plead guilty to the charge, and was placed in a drug rehabilitation program.[1]

One year later, Daniels was hired by the Topeka Sizzlers in the Continental Basketball League (CBA). Although he averaged 16 points a game, he was suspended after only 29 games for failure to participate in his drug rehabilitation program. Given another chance to play, he went to Auckland, New Zealand. Again he played outstandingly well, averaging 27 points a game, but was cut from the team in May 1988 for a drinking problem. He had been purportedly drinking a case of beer per day.[3] Sweet Pea returned to the United States and tried out for two other CBA teams (Quad Cities and

Albany); however, he was cut from both after very short, unremarkable stints.

In May 1989 Lloyd Daniels was shot three times in the chest and neck during an $8 drug dispute outside his grandmother's home in Queens.[1] Although critically injured, he recovered and returned to the city basketball courts where his mythical status lived on.

Though talented, Daniels lacked structure and motivation. He had little self discipline, few positive role models he would listen too, and was unprepared for the harsh realities of life off the basketball court. Drugs, alcohol, and indifference took their toll. The promising "big money" athletic career plummeted. He is lucky to have escaped with his life.

Lloyd Daniels, a legend in his own mind, has been in drug rehabilitation programs between two and five times, depending on who's story you believe. Despite the treatment programs, no one believes any longer that he will be able to stay away from drugs. The cliques and circles where drugs are most prevalent are the same places where he is most revered.

Lloyd Daniels applied for the N.B.A. draft but no teams were interested in him.[3] He now plays in the United States Basketball League (USBL). The league, which plays a 20-game June-July schedule, refers to itself as the "league of opportunity." According to some reports, Sweet Pea is making "the least of his opportunities" there.[2] Without the inner resources to live the healthy, disciplined life required in professional sports, Sweet Pea will forever be relegated to the streets or minor leagues where hype, flattery, and praise abound, but where no one takes him seriously. His friends still come out to see him play and continue to believe he's a franchise maker whose time will come. NBA scouts also come to see him play, but now mostly out of curiosity, wondering "what if?"

Environment of Exception

Although Lloyd Daniels was the victim of a hostile environment and vicious educational and social systems, Daniels also failed himself. Unlike many of his peers, he had chances, many chances. Although uneducated, he was not stupid. His ability to understand

and play out the intricate and complicated strategies of fast paced basketball attest to that.

Lloyd Daniels' inability to manage the increasing demands and responsibilities of college and professional sports can be traced to one fact: that he was never held accountable for his actions. He did not learn what most of us learn at an early age: that there are consequences for unacceptable or inappropriate behavior. No matter what rules he broke, he was given another chance. His shortcomings were dismissed or ignored, and his basketball talent afforded him special considerations. He was raised and sacrificed in an "environment of exception."

For a select group of highly talented student athletes, this environment is often unconsciously fostered and nurtured in junior high school where the first signs of superior physical skills are observed. These unique individuals are more agile, have better hand-eye coordination, and are able to jump higher and run faster than their peers. They are usually bigger, taller, and stronger than their age-mates. Psychologically, these individuals are taken out of the normal student population and put on a special course. Teachers, peers, friends, and relatives treat them with reverence. Local recognition spreads to state recognition.[4] They slowly become exempt from many of the rules and regulations that directly affect other students, and as they move from high school to college, they expect this preferential treatment to continue.

In many cases it does, but when the expectations of the elite student athlete and the realities of social life clash, a very confused, bitter, frightened, and often depressed young adult can emerge. Student athletes who are unwilling or unable to adjust to the new realities must then find other ways to get their needs met. Far too often, alcohol and other drugs of abuse are used to accomplish this end. Drugs are used in an attempt to mask or escape the pain and uncertainties of the new setting.

Authors note: Lloyd Daniel's trouble-plagued route to the NBA took a curious turn when he signed a two-year contract with the San Antonio Spurs on July 21, 1992. Daniels joins first year coach, Jerry Tarkanian, who recruited Sweet Pea when the coach was at UNLV.

Whether Daniels has learned enough from his past mistakes to take advantage of this unique opportunity, only time will tell.

Non-Performance Enhancing Drug Use

Student athletes are acutely aware of the importance of a healthy mind and body. Why then, would they use illicit drugs that are known to be destructive to their mental and physical well-being?

Student athletes, like everyone else, use drugs to feel good. They use drugs when their emotional needs are not being met. Drugs are taken to alter their perception of reality, and they are taken in an attempt to escape from the daily stresses that accompany the dual role they perform in.

High school and college is a time when young athletes are expected to learn, process information, train, and perform. As a student, you are also motivated to question and challenge your longstanding beliefs, ideas, and attitudes. For many high school and college athletes, this learning and analyzing process leads to experimentation with alcohol and other drugs.

Student athletes are raised and nurtured in a culture where the use of performance aids is commonplace. They see that it's acceptable to jump-start the day with coffee, buffer the day with cigarettes, valium, and alcohol, and end the day with a sedative to relax or get to sleep. The use of these socially accepted performance enhancers fosters the student athlete's mentality and appetite for drugs to ease mental and physical anguish and achieve goals.

Stress Producing Factors

Student athletes are under tremendous amounts of pressure. In fact, they live and survive in an environment of pressure and uncertainty. There is pressure to succeed and pressure to win. This pressure comes from two sources: the athletes's strong inner drive; and the pressure placed on schools, colleges, athletic administrations, and coaches, to win. Whether voiced or not, the pressure to win is easily transferred to the athlete.

Performance Enhancing Drug Use

The marriage between athletics and drugs has been around longer than any of us have been alive. In the third century B.C. Homer described athletes who took mushrooms to make them faster and stronger.[5] Later, Greek athletes were said to depend on root extracts, and the Egyptians, on rose tips to bolster their athletic prowess. This need for athletic perfection has continued unabated. In the 1900s runners used nitroglycerine to thin the blood, increasing the amount of blood pumped to the heart and thereby increasing the body's oxygen supply.[5]

Still, it is difficult for most people to understand the intense competitive nature of some student athletes and how motivated, compulsive, and focused they can be when pursuing high performance and recognition. Some young athletes believe they are immortal. They are primarily concerned with victory now and don't give much thought to the potential dangers of certain drugs five to ten years down the road.

Sports medicine, exercise physiology, sports psychology, and other disciplines have shown student athletes how to enhance athletic performance while safeguarding their health. It should be no surprise then, that some athletes resort to pharmacological agents to gain an extra edge in competitive sports.[4] Most competitive athletes don't sacrifice, train, or perform for their health. They have a very specific agenda; to win. The legalities, ethics, and morals regarding fair play are understood, but often they are not prime concerns when striving for superior performance.

Victory doesn't have to be a state title, regional or NCAA championship, or an Olympic gold medal. It can be small and personal, such as winning the local 10k race, the fraternity championship, or setting a new personal best in weight lifting. If athletes of any stature with a "win at all cost" attitude believe their competitor is using a technique or aid that gives them an advantage, they will seek it out and use it too.

Factors for Success

Fortunately, most student athletes avoid illegal aids and shortcuts, and stay away from illicit performance enhancing drugs. They achieve their goals through planning, long and intense training sessions, proper nutrition, and adequate rest. Throughout athletic history, these methods have been effective in setting record times and winning gold medals, college scholarships, and professional contracts. By using this tried and true system, individual and team records will continue to be broken. The reasons for the continued advancement in sports achievements are many. They include:[6]

1. Selection from a larger and healthier population
2. Better coaching and training methods
3. Improved facilities
4. Technological improvements in equipment design
5. Better nutrition and medical treatment

Although not all student athletes are created equally, dedication, commitment, and proper training can develop your natural abilities so that you can accomplish your goals and perform at levels you desire. [6]

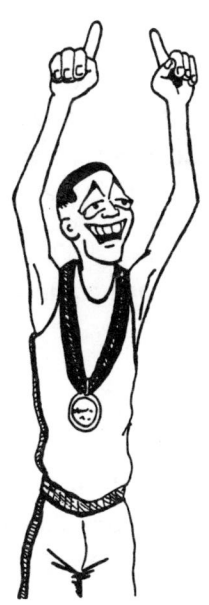

Summary

Media exposes, forever highlight the drug problems of former and present student athletes. This clearly shows that athletic ability offers no special immunity to drug abuse. Even streetwise, superbly conditioned and trained "super athletes" are as vulnerable to substance abuse as are other members of society.[4]

Competitive athletics is staged in an environment where the rewards for winning can be enormous and where those less fortunate, despite their best efforts, are often forgotten. I understand the obvious conflicts and problems associated with such a system. Especially since most of your life you're told that it doesn't matter whether you win or lose, but how you play the game. However, drug use to soothe the ego, calm fears, or eliminate an unfair advantage you *believe* your competitors have will not change the system. It only makes your situation worse.

If you're going to reach your full potential and achieve your goals in the classroom and on the athletic field, you should be aware of the physical and psychological problems that accompany drug use. Illicit drugs and treatments are dangerous. They can cut short your academic and athletic career and, quite possibly, your life. In the athletic arena there are no quick fixes, magic formulas, or shortcuts. If there were, there would be no need for competition because everyone would be number one, and it wouldn't mean a thing. So you see, it's the same now as it has always been: it takes planning, dedication, commitment; blood, sweat, and tears, to be successful. A healthy mind and body is essential to achieve top performance.

Playing with drugs is the one game you cannot win!

References

1. Scorecard: The Sad Tale Of Sweet Pea. Sports Illustrated, May 22, 1989.
2. Looney DS: Legend or Myth? Sports Illustrated, July 8, 1991 p.40.
3. McKinley JC: A Star Once, Felled First By Drugs, Now Bullets. The New York Times, May 13, 1989 p.1.

2. Looney, p.41
4. Wadler GI, Hainline B: Drugs and the Athlete. Philadelphia, F.A. Davis Company 1989.
5. Dealy Jr. FX: Win at any Cost. The Sell Out of College Athletics. 1990 Birch Lane Press Book, Carol Publishing Group.
6. Williams MH: Beyond Training: How Athletes Enhance Performance Legally and Illegally. 1989 Leisure Press. Champaign, IL

Index

A

Accuracy of drug testing, 49
Acromegaly, 60
Addiction, 22, 23, 40, 76, 79
Advertising, 73
Aggressiveness, 40
Agitation, 23, 38, 75
AIDS, 63
Alcohol, 6
    and carbohydrates, 11
    and myths, 6, 13
    and problem drinking, 14
    and sedatives, 85
    and sobering process, 12
    and wine coolers, 12
    blood alcohol concentrations, 9
    case vignette for, 16
    drinking situations, 11
    effect on females, 12
    effects of, 6, 7, 8
    legal rights, 10
    toll free hotline, 16
Alcoholism, 14
Alcohol dehydrogenase, 12
Amphetamines, 78
    athletes use of, reasons for, 79
    clinical uses, 78
    commonly abused, 78
    effects of, 79, 80, 81
    on performance, 81
    street names, 78
Anabolic steroids, 33
    and athletic performance, 36, 37
    athletes use of, reasons for, 34
    case vignette for, 33
    effects of, 37-40
    effect on children, 37
    effect on females, 38
    legal rights, 40
Animal growth hormone. See Human growth hormone.
Anorexia, 20
Anxiety, 23
    effects of depressants on, 84
Anabolic-androgenic steroids. See Anabolic steroids.
Astma medications, 76, 81
Autologous blood transfusion, 62-63

B

Barbiturates, effects of, 83
Benson and Hedges, 73
Benzodiazepines, effects of, 83
Bias, Len, 1-2
Blood alcohol concentrations, 9
Blood doping, 62
    athletes use of, reasons for, 62
    effects of, 63
    procedure for, 62-63
    sports where used, 62
    legal rights, 64

C

Caffeine, 69
    athletes use of, reasons for, 69
    drug testing for, 55
    effects of, 69
    legal status, 69
Carbohydrates, in alcohol, 11

Central nervous system, response of, to,
- amphetamines, 78
- caffeine, 69
- chewing tobacco, 72

Cigarettes, See Nicotine.
Civil liberties, See Drug testing.
Cocaine, 18
- addiction to, 19, 22
- case vignette for, 20
- death from, 1-2, 20
- definition, 18
- effects of, 20, 21
- history, 18
- in sports, 19
- main actions of, 20

Coffee, See Caffeine.
Corticosteroids, 35
Cough preparations, See Stimulants
Cravings, 23
Croudip, David, 20

D

Daniels, Lloyd, 87-89
Decongestants. See Ephedrine.
DeMont, Rick, 77
Depressants, 83
- and alcohol, 85-86
- athletes use of, reasons for, 84
- clinical uses, 83
- effects of, 84-86
- street names, 83

Diuretics, 50
Drug testing, 44
- accuracy of, 49
- civil liberties, 44
- consent, 44
- controversy over, 44
- for cocaine, 50
- methods of, 47
- rationale for, 45
- sources of error in, 49

Drug testing policies
- of NCAA, 51-53
- of USOC, 51-53

E

Endurance athletes
- amphetamines and, 78-79
- blood doping and, 62
- caffeine and, 69
- erythropoietin and, 64

Ephedrine, 76
- clinical uses, 76
- drug testing for, 81
- effects of, 77
- in over-the-counter medications, 76, 81

Erythropoietin, 64
- athletes use of, reasons for, 65
- clinical uses, 64
- definition, 64
- effects on performance, 65
- negative effects, 66

Eye-hand coordination, 7, 28, 84-85

F

False-negative, 49
False-positive, 49
Fatigue
- caffeine use for, 69
- stimulants use for, 80

Female reproductive system, effects of anabolic steroids on, 38

G

Gas chromatography-mass spectroscopy (GC/MS), 48
Gender factors
  in alcohol metabolism, 12
Growth hormone. See human growth hormone
Gymnasts
  use of depressants, 84
  use of amphetamines, 79
Gynecomastia, 37

H

Hair analysis, 50
Hashish, 26
Hemp plant, 25
Hemoglobin
  relation to blood doping, 62
hGH See human growth hormone.
Hormones
  effect of anabolic steroids on, 37-38
Homologous blood transfusion, 62-63
Hotline, toll-free, 16
Human growth hormone, 58
  athletes use of, reasons for, 59
  clinical uses, 58
  cost of, 59
  definition, 58
  effects of, 60

I

International Olympic Committee (IOC)
  banning of stimulants, 76
  policy on marijuana, 31
Irritability, 64, 69

J

Johnson, Ben, 35

K

Kimble, Bruce, 16

L

Liver
  effects of alcohol, 7
  effects of anabolic steroids, 38
Loose-leaf tobacco, 72
Lung cancer, nicotine and, 74

M

Male reproductive system, effects of anabolic steroids on, 37-38
Marijuana, 24
  and psychological dependence, 27-28
  as hashish, 26
  case vignette for, 24
  clinical uses, 28
  definition, 25
  effects of, 27-28
  legal rights, 31
  myths, 29
Marsee, Sean, 70-71
Metabolism, 12
Myers, Angel, 33

N

Nasal decongestants, 76
National Collegiate Athletic Association (NCAA)
  drugs banned by, 52
  drug testing protocol, 35, 51-53
Nicotine,
  addiction to, 71

and advertising, 73-74
and passive inhalation, 74-75
athletes use of, reasons for, 73
case vignette, 70-71
effects of, 74-75
in smokeless tobacco, 72
role of in tobacco, 72
Nitrosamines, 74

O

Olympic Games
    drug scandals, 33, 35
Oxygen
    relation to blood doping, 62

P

Pistol shooting
    effect of depressants on, 84
Plug, tobacco, 72
Privacy, issue of,
    See Drug Testing
Problem drinking. See Alcohol.
Pseudoephedrine. See Ephedrine
Psychomotor stimulant drugs
    banned list, 53

R

Red blood cells.
See Blood doping.
Rifle shooting
    effects of depressants on, 84
Rogers, Don, 1-2

S

Sedatives. See Depressants.
Smokeless tobacco. See Nicotine.
Steroids. See Anabolic Steroids.
Stimulants, 68

Stress
    and athletes, 91
    drug use and, 90
Sudden death, 20

T

Testosterone, 36, 55
Tetrahydrocannabinol (THC), 25-26
Tobacco. See Nicotine.
Transfusion
    autologous, 62-63
    homologous, 62-63

U

United States Olympic Committee (USOC)
    drugs banned by, 52
    drug testing protocol, 51-53
United States Tobacco Company, 73
Urine drug testing, 47

V

Valium, 83
Virginia Slims, 73

W

Wine coolers, 12
Winning
    drug use and, 91
    pressure for, 91

About the Author

Marvin L. Sims is a sports counselor in the department of Sports Medicine at the University of Iowa Hospitals and Clinics in Iowa City, Iowa. He specializes in counseling for student athletes.

Born in Sedalia, Missouri, Marvin spent six years in the United States Air Force as an Air Traffic Control Operator. He moved to Iowa City, Iowa in 1972 and since has received his undergraduate degree(BA) and a masters degree (MSW) in Social Work from the University of Iowa. Marvin is licensed by the Iowa Board of Substance Abuse Certification (IBSAC), and he has an independent practice as a psychotherapist. In his spare time, he enjoys weight training, and biking, and relishes the challenges of one- on-one basketball.

What Every Student Athlete Must Know About Drugs The Handbook

Marvin L. Sims, MSW, CAC

ORDER FORM

Name _____

Street _____

City _____ State _____ Zip _____

Copies   X $10.95   EACH = $ _____
Shipping = $ _____
Total = $ _____

Add $3.00 shipping for one copy
$4.00 for two copies
$5.00 for three or more

Please make all checks or money orders payable to:
Marvin L. Sims
1265 Melrose Ave.
Iowa City, IA 52246

Allow 2-4 weeks for delivery

What Every Student Athlete Must Know About Drugs The Handbook

Marvin L. Sims, MSW, CAC

ORDER FORM

Name _____

Street _____

City _____ State _____ Zip _____

Copies X $10.95   EACH = $ _____
Shipping = $ _____
Total = $ _____

Add $3.00 shipping for one copy
$4.00 for two copies
$5.00 for three or more

Please make all checks or money orders payable to:
Marvin L. Sims
1265 Melrose Ave.
Iowa City, IA 52246

Allow 2-4 weeks for delivery